DIGESTIVE DISEASES – RESEARCH AND CLINICAL DEVELOPMENTS

COLITIS

CAUSES, DIAGNOSIS AND TREATMENT

DIGESTIVE DISEASES – RESEARCH AND CLINICAL DEVELOPMENTS

Additional books and e-books in this series can be found on Nova's website under the Series tab.

DIGESTIVE DISEASES – RESEARCH AND CLINICAL DEVELOPMENTS

COLITIS

CAUSES, DIAGNOSIS AND TREATMENT

SOREN GARCIA
EDITOR

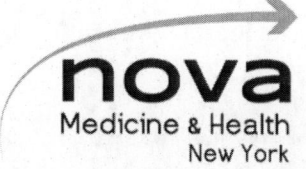

Copyright © 2019 by Nova Science Publishers, Inc.

All rights reserved. No part of this book may be reproduced, stored in a retrieval system or transmitted in any form or by any means: electronic, electrostatic, magnetic, tape, mechanical photocopying, recording or otherwise without the written permission of the Publisher.

We have partnered with Copyright Clearance Center to make it easy for you to obtain permissions to reuse content from this publication. Simply navigate to this publication's page on Nova's website and locate the "Get Permission" button below the title description. This button is linked directly to the title's permission page on copyright.com. Alternatively, you can visit copyright.com and search by title, ISBN, or ISSN.

For further questions about using the service on copyright.com, please contact:
Copyright Clearance Center
Phone: +1-(978) 750-8400   Fax: +1-(978) 750-4470   E-mail: info@copyright.com.

NOTICE TO THE READER

The Publisher has taken reasonable care in the preparation of this book, but makes no expressed or implied warranty of any kind and assumes no responsibility for any errors or omissions. No liability is assumed for incidental or consequential damages in connection with or arising out of information contained in this book. The Publisher shall not be liable for any special, consequential, or exemplary damages resulting, in whole or in part, from the readers' use of, or reliance upon, this material. Any parts of this book based on government reports are so indicated and copyright is claimed for those parts to the extent applicable to compilations of such works.

Independent verification should be sought for any data, advice or recommendations contained in this book. In addition, no responsibility is assumed by the Publisher for any injury and/or damage to persons or property arising from any methods, products, instructions, ideas or otherwise contained in this publication.

This publication is designed to provide accurate and authoritative information with regard to the subject matter covered herein. It is sold with the clear understanding that the Publisher is not engaged in rendering legal or any other professional services. If legal or any other expert assistance is required, the services of a competent person should be sought. FROM A DECLARATION OF PARTICIPANTS JOINTLY ADOPTED BY A COMMITTEE OF THE AMERICAN BAR ASSOCIATION AND A COMMITTEE OF PUBLISHERS.

Additional color graphics may be available in the e-book version of this book.

Library of Congress Cataloging-in-Publication Data

ISBN: 978-1-53616-631-6

Published by Nova Science Publishers, Inc. † New York

CONTENTS

Preface		vii
Chapter 1	Infections of Clostridium Difficile *L. Palcová, A. Lesňáková and B. Matúšková*	1
Chapter 2	Sulfate Source and Its Role in the Development of Colitis *Ivan Kushkevych*	19
Chapter 3	Helminth Therapy: A Promising Biotherapeutic Approach for Autoimmune Colitis *Kalyan Goswami, Vishal Khatri, Nitin Amdare, Namdev Togre and Priyanka Bhoj*	75
Index		131
Related Nova Publications		137

PREFACE

Clostridium difficile and its toxin-producing strains are the most common causative agents of *Clostridium difficile* infections. It is an inflammatory bowel disease predominantly caused by prior antibiotic treatment. The use of broad spectrum antibiotics suppresses bacterial intestinal microflora and causes overgrowth of the *Clostridium difficile*, and often occurs in immunocompromised, older and polymorbid patients.

Following this, the authors discuss inflammatory bowel disease (including ulcerative colitis), a complex, multifactorial disease of unknown etiology. Intestinal sulfate-reducing bacteria, especially Desuflovibrio, are often found in the intestines and feces of people and animals with inflammatory bowel disease.

Of late, the incidence of autoimmune colitis both in adults and children has been progressively increasing globally. The efficacy of conventional therapeutic measures is questionably limited due to short-term immunosuppressive effect along with possible serious side effects. As such, the authors present evidence from epidemiological studies that has demonstrated an inverse relationship between the occurrence of parasitic diseases and various autoimmune pathologies.

Chapter 1 – Introduction. *Clostridium difficile* (CD) and its toxin producing strains are the most common causative agents of *Clostridium difficile* infections (CDI). It is an inflammatory bowel disease mostly caused by prior antibiotic treatment. The use of broad spectrum antibiotics suppresses bacterial intestinal microflora and cause overgrowth of the genus CD. It often occurs in immunocompromised, older and polymorbid patients. Despite intensive research into new drugs that are effective in treating CDI, treatment is still a major problem, especially given the high probability of recurrence and resistance to treatment. Aim. The aim of this study is to retrospectively evaluate the presence of CD toxins in fecal samples from patients with antibiotic-associated diarrhea, examined in the Institute of Clinical Microbiology, Central Military Hospital SNP - Faculty Hospital, Ružomberok (CMH SNP Rbk FH) for the year 2018. Based on the authors' chosen criteria, the authors compared individual risk factors in given patients. Method. Stool samples from patients with antibiotic-associated diarrhea were tested in the Institute of Clinical Microbiology, CMH SNP Rbk-FH. Since the metabolic enzyme glutamate dehydrogenase (GDH), which produces CD strains, is considered a screening marker for the presence of CD in fecal samples, all samples were initially tested for GDH. Detection of GDH in stool samples is based on the immunochromatographic principle. If positive, toxins should be determined. All these tests were commercially available diagnostic tests. The authors evaluated their criteria in all toxin positive patients: age, sex, ward, diagnosis, stool count, temperature incidence, increased CRP, leukocytosis, increased albumin levels, increased creatinine levels, patient immobility, type of antibiotic therapy prior to CDI symptoms, occurrence of abdominal surgeries, oncological history, subsequent treatment of clostridial enterocolitis and the number of possible relapses. The Results. From 01 January 2018 to 31 December 2018, 382 stools were screened for GDH in the Institute of Clinical Microbiology. Of these, 190 stools were GDH positive (49.74 percent). These samples were examined for the presence of toxins. Of these, 87 stools (45.79 percent) were toxin positive. The occurrence of toxin A was detected in 14 samples (16.10 percent), toxin B was detected in 7 samples (8.10 percent). The incidence of both A and B toxins at the same time was the most numerous, accounting for 66 samples (75.80 percent). Conclusion. Based on the authors' findings from the analysis of selected criteria and the assessment of risk factors, they can conclude that in older polymorbid patients, CDI treatment can be prolonged with relatively frequent relapses, as described in a 75-year-old patient with six CDI recurrences. The ATLAS predictive scoring mortality system helps to predict a disease prognosis, relapses and mortality. Prevention means the appropriate and targeted antibiotic therapy, following the hygiene and epidemiology measures, taking probiotics along with antibiotic treatment and opting for a highly effective fidaxomicin therapy.

Chapter 2 - Inflammatory bowel disease (IBD), including ulcerative colitis (UC), is a complex multifactorial disease of unknown etiology. Intestinal sulfate-reducing bacteria (SRB), especially *Desuflovibrio* genus are often found in the intestines and feces of people and animals with IBD. One of the main roles in the development of UC among other factors can also be the species of this genus. These bacteria use sulfate as a terminal electron acceptor and organic compounds as an electron donor in their metabolisms. This fact leads us to the conclusion that sulfate present in the daily diet plays an important role in the development of bowel disease. Sulfate is present mainly in the following food commodities: i) some breads, soya flour, dried fruits, brassicas, and sausages; ii) as well as some beers, ciders, and wines. These data indicate that sulfate intake is highly dependent on diet. Literature data indicates that sulfate level present in diet among people living in more developed countries consume over 16.6 mmole of sulfate per day. It should be noted the role of sulfite present in food since it can also be consumed by SRB. The complexity of sulfate metabolism can be overviewed by data that focuses on the intestinal environment containing different concentrations of hydrogen sulfide produced by SRB. According to the fact mentioned above, this chapter is dealing with issues concerning sulfate present in different food commodities and the intestinal environment affecting mainly SRB. These issues are explained by literature data indicating the role of sulfate in the intestines of animals, including humans. The data present in this chapter can be used to better explain of IBD and improve therapeutic strategies.

Chapter 3 - Of late, the incidence of autoimmune colitis both in adults and children has been progressively increasing globally. The efficacy of conventional therapeutic measures is questionably limited due to short-term immunosuppressive effect along with possible serious side effects. Evidence from epidemiological studies has demonstrated an inverse relationship between the occurrence of parasitic diseases and various autoimmune pathologies. Co-evolution of parasitic nematodes with humans possibly led to a positive selection pressure favoring a more tolerogenic immune response as an effective strategy of immune-evasion favoring long-term patency of parasitism. These immunomodulatory strategies have provided a significant cue for an alternative therapeutic approach. As proof of this premise, recent evidence has established a platform for the emergence of helminth-therapy as a promising alternative bio-therapeutics for colitis and other immune-mediated disorders. Studies in experimental models of colitis have shown that live/attenuated worms or their eggs or the soluble and/or excretory-secretory products of helminths have definitive therapeutic potential. Several clinical trials have also been conducted in colitis patients aiming to replicate the success of such experimental studies. However, utilization of live/attenuated worms or the crude products derived from them can cause serious complications with obvious ethical concerns, hence rendering these attempts controversial. Therefore, it seems more rational to explore and exploit specific immunomodulatory proteins from parasites having a more selective effect against colitis. Outcomes from the experimental studies that identified and demonstrated the efficacy of the use of certain recombinant parasitic proteins against ulcerative colitis have opened a new vista for developing helminth derived biotherapeutics against colitis. There is a definitive need to focus on this aspect for a better insight to utilize this novel therapeutic venture effectively and safely to resolve a very socially relevant health problem of recent times.

In: Colitis: Causes, Diagnosis and Treatment   ISBN: 978-1-53616-631-6
Editor: Soren Garcia   © 2019 Nova Science Publishers, Inc.

Chapter 1

INFECTIONS OF CLOSTRIDIUM DIFFICILE

L. Palcová[1,], A. Lesňáková[2,4] and B. Matúšková[3,5]*

[1]Institute of Clinical Microbiology, Central Military
Hospital SNP-FN, Ružomberok, Slovakia
[2]Clinic Infectology, Central Military
Hospital SNP-FH Ružomberok, Slovakia
[3]Clinic of Anaesthesiology and Intensive Central Military Hospital
SNP-FH Ružomberok, Slovakia
[4]Faculty of Health, Catholic Univerzity, Ružomberok, Slovakia
[5]St. Elisabeth University of Health Care and Social Work,
Bratislava, Slovakia

ABSTRACT

Introduction

Clostridium difficile (CD) and its toxin producing strains are the most common causative agents of *Clostridium difficile* infections (CDI).

---

[*] Ccorresponding Author: Mgr. Lenka Palcová, Institute of Clinical Microbiology Central Military Hospital SNP-FN, gen .M. Vesela 21, 034 26 Ružomberok, E-mail: palcoval@uvn.sk.

It is an inflammatory bowel disease mostly caused by prior antibiotic treatment. The use of broad spectrum antibiotics suppresses bacterial intestinal microflora and cause overgrowth of the genus CD. It often occurs in immunocompromised, older and polymorbid patients. Despite intensive research into new drugs that are effective in treating CDI, treatment is still a major problem, especially given the high probability of recurrence and resistance to treatment.

Aim

The aim of this study is to retrospectively evaluate the presence of CD toxins in fecal samples from patients with antibiotic-associated diarrhea, examined in the Institute of Clinical Microbiology, Central Military Hospital SNP - Faculty Hospital, Ružomberok (CMH SNP Rbk FH) for the year 2018. Based on our chosen criteria, we compared individual risk factors in given patients.

Method

Stool samples from patients with antibiotic-associated diarrhea were tested in the Institute of Clinical Microbiology, CMH SNP Rbk-FH.Since the metabolic enzyme glutamate dehydrogenase (GDH), which produces CD strains, is considered a screening marker for the presence of CD in fecal samples, all samples were initially tested for GDH. Detection of GDH in stool samples is based on the immunochromatographic principle. If positive, toxins should be determined. All these tests were commercially available diagnostic tests. We evaluated our criteria in all toxin positive patients: age, sex, ward, diagnosis, stool count, temperature incidence, increased CRP, leukocytosis, increased albumin levels, increased creatinine levels, patient immobility, type of antibiotic therapy prior to CDI symptoms, occurrence of abdominal surgeries, oncological history, subsequent treatment of clostridial enterocolitis and the number of possible relapses.

The Results

From 01 January 2018 to 31 December 2018, 382 stools were screened for GDH in the Institute of Clinical Microbiology. Of these, 190 stools were GDH positive (49.74 percent). These samples were examined for the presence of toxins. Of these, 87 stools (45.79 percent) were toxin positive. The occurrence of toxin A was detected in 14 samples (16.10

percent), toxin B was detected in 7 samples (8.10 percent). The incidence of both A and B toxins at the same time was the most numerous, accounting for 66 samples (75.80 percent).

Conclusion

Based on our findings from the analysis of selected criteria and the assessment of risk factors, we can conclude that in older polymorbid patients, CDI treatment can be prolonged with relatively frequent relapses, as described in a 75-year-old patient with six CDI recurrences. The ATLAS predictive scoring mortality system helps to predict a disease prognosis, relapses and mortality. Prevention means the appropriate and targeted antibiotic therapy, following the hygiene and epidemiology measures, taking probiotics along with antibiotic treatment and opting for a highly effective fidaxomicin therapy.

Keywords: Clostridium difficile, antibiotic treatment, risk factors, recurrence

INTRODUCTION

Clostridium difficile is a gram-positive anaerobic bacterium that is commonly found in nature, in surface water and with varying frequencies in the digestive tract of humans and animals. Under unfavorable conditions, metabolically inactive forms - spores that are thermoresistant, resist physical effects, also resist commonly used disinfectants. These factors are closely related to the incidence of nosocomial infections. The pathogenicity of this microbe is due to its ability to form highly potent exotoxins that are considered to be major factors in virulence. *Clostridium difficile* infections – CD is are closely related to antibiotic use and show a wide range of clinical manifestations ranging from mild diarrhea through pseudomembrane colitis, sepsis to toxic megacolon. This type of infection is a treatment-related increase in health costs, as well as high mortality and frequent occurrence of remissions are a global health care problem (Guh, A.Y., et al., 2018).

ETIOPATHOGENESIS

The disease is most commonly associated with treatment with broad spectrum antibiotics. These eliminate the physiological intestinal flora. CDI arises when two conditions are met, namely: loss of intestinal microflora and infection with toxigenic strains of Clostridium difficile. These strains produce two kinds of toxins. Toxin A (TcdA) belongs to enterotoxins. Its mechanism of action is to damage the cells of the intestinal epithelium, resulting in the accumulation of fluid in the intestine, affecting the formation of watery, often hemorrhagic diarrhea. Toxin B (TcdB) acts on cytotoxic cells of the intestine, causing necrosis of infected cells. Numerous, typical maple ulcerations covered with membrane of are found on the colon mucosa during colonoscopic examination. The action of toxin B on smooth muscle and vegetative nerves in the colon wall slows down peristalsis and ileum development. Such damage may result in intestinal perforation. The terminal stage of the disease is characterized by an enormous distension of the colon (megacolon) and a gradual loss of the barrier function of the intestinal mucosa with subsequent development of the septic state. The most common etiological agent of the septic state is the gram-negative bacteria, such as the intestinal microflora, which penetrate the surrounding structures through perforation (McDonald LC, et al., 2018). The clinical picture of diarrhea is very variable. From mild to moderate diarrhea with no general symptoms, to pseudomembranous enterocolitis with severe or even fulminant course. More serious forms of the disease are accompanied by abdominal pain, meteorism, gradual disappearance of intestinal peristalsis, which leads to the development of the ileum (Jarčuška, P., et al., 2015).

RISK FACTORS

Other risk factors besides the antibiotics most commonly associated with CDI (fluoroquinolones, cephalosporins III.generation, clindamycin and penicillins) are higher patient age, overall immobility, abdominal surgery, immunodeficiency, organ transplantation, oncological status with chemotherapy, suppression gastric acid and other other civilization diseases (diabetes melitus).

EPIDEMIOLOGY

On the basis of the "Epidemiological Situation and Activity of Epidemiology Departments in the Slovak Republic in 2018", the most common biological material in nosocomial infections was Clostridium difficile in 20.9 percent. By comparing the number of CDIs in Slovakia with the incidence in the Central Military Hospital in Ružomberok, we found that their abundance in the Central Military Hospital Ružomberok is statistically significantly lower than the observed average in Slovakia, which is at a significance level of 0.05.

THERAPY

In less serious cases, if the patient's condition allows it we interrupt antibiotics therapy and we start with all necessary actions to improve clinical status of the patient. For medical treatment of patients with not seriously CDI these antibiotics are most commonly used: fidaxomicin, metronidazol, teikoplanin, vankomycin. Profylactical probiotic therapy significantly reduces by 54% occurrence of diarrhea during antibiotic treatment. Fecal transplantation is officially recommended treatment method for treatment of multiple CDI recurrences with high percentage of efficiency which overcomes existing antibiotics treatment (Polák, P., a spol., 2015). Fidaxomicin (trade names Dificid, Dificlir, and previously OPT-80 and PAR-101) is the first member of a class of narrow spectrum macrolids antibiotic drugs and is registered only for CDI treatment. It is not absorbed from GIT so there are not systematic side effects.

Fidaxomicin binds to and prevents movement of the "switch regions" of bacterial RNA polymerase. Switch motion occurs during the opening and closing of the DNA:RNA clamp, a process that occurs throughout RNA transcription but is especially important in the opening of double-stranded DNA during the initiation of transcription. It has minimal systemic absorption and a narrow spectrum of activity; it is active against Gram-positive bacteria, especially *clostridium*. The minimal inhibitory concentration (MIC) range for *Clostridium difficile* (ATCC 700057) is 0.03–0.25 µg/mL (Srivastava, A., et al., 2011).

OBJECTIVE

The main goal of this study is to retrospectively evaluate the incidence of Clostridium difficile in stool samples of patients with postantibiotic diarrhea, examined in the Institute of Clinical Microbiology, SNP-FN Central Military Hospital, Ružomberok in year 2018. Based on our criteria, we compared individual risk factors in 382 cases.

METHODS

Our study retrospectively evaluated stool samples of patients examined at the Institute of Clinical Microbiology, SNP-FN Central Military Hospital, Ružomberok during the period from 01.01.2018 to 31.12.2018. The study was prepared with the consent of the Ethics Committee, SNP-FN Central Military Hospital, Ružomberok.

Collection of Biological Material

For microbiological examination of samples for the presence of Clostridium difficile, samples of approximately 2 ml should be taken into a sterile container. The stool sample must be examined within two hours after collection because the toxins are relatively unstable and rapidly degraded. If the sample cannot be transported to the laboratory immediately after collection, it can be stored at refrigerator temperature (5 °C) for 48 hours. For long-term sample storage, the sample should be frozen at -70 °C.

In the Institute of Clinical Microbiology, Central Military Hospital SNP-FN, Ružomberok, the following laboratory diagnostic procedure for the detection of Clostridium difficile is determined:

1. Determination of glutamatedehydrogenase
2. Determination of toxins A / B

Determination of Glutamatedehydrogenase

Since the metabolic enzyme glutamatedehydrogenase GDH that produces Clostridium difficile strains is considered a screening marker for the presence of *Clostridium difficile* in stool samples. Its diagnosis is based on the immunochromatography principle. All stool samples were examined with the VEDA-LAB GDH-CHECK-1 diagnostic kit. Subsequently, positive samples were further examined for the presence of toxins.

Determination of A / B toxins

The presence of toxin A or B was determined by the VEDA-LAB DUO TOXIN A + B-CHECK-1 assay. The assay is based on the immunochromatographic principle. It detects the presence of toxin A or B, or both.

During the period from 01.01.2018 to 31.12.2018 the Institute of Clinical Microbiology, Central Military Hospital SNP-FN, Ružomberok received 382 samples to detect GDH. From this amount 192 samples were GDH negative (50,26%) and 190 samples were GDH positive (49,74%). Positive samples were examined for presence of toxins. 103 samples from this were negative (54,21%) and 87 were positive (45,79%). Toxin A was proven in 14 samples (16,10%) and toxin B in 7 (8,10%) samples. Presence of both toxins A,B together was the largest group of samples and we detected them in 66 samples (75,80%).

Positive patients were evaluated by the standard criteria used in the Institute of Clinical Microbiology, Central Military Hospital SNP-FN, Ružomberok.

RESULTS

From January 1, 2018 to December 31, 2018, 382 stools samples were examined for the presence of GDH at the Institute of Clinical Microbiology. Of these, 192 GDH stools were negative (50.26 percent). And 190 stools samples were positive for GDH (49.74 percent). Subsequently, 190 stools samples were examined for the presence of toxins. Of the 190 stools samples, 103 samples represented negativity (54.21 percent) and 87 positivity (45.79 percent). The presence of toxin A was detected in 14 samples (16.10 percent), toxin B in 7 samples (8.10 percent). At the same time, the incidence of both toxins A and B was the highest, accounting for 66 samples (75.80 percent). Patients whose presence of toxins was confirmed in stool samples were evaluated according to our criteria.

Evaluation of Results by Age and Gender

Of the 87 patients who were found to be toxins, women accounted for 59, which is 67.82 percent. Men represented a smaller group of 28, which is 32.18 percent. The average age for women was 74 years, with the youngest woman being 31 years old and the oldest woman 105 years old. For men, the average age was 70 years, with the youngest man being 33 and the oldest man 87.

Evaluation of Results by Department

Out of a total of 87 patients, up to 29 samples for the diagnosis of Clostridium difficile in stool samples were ordained from the after-treatment department. Twenty-four samples were collected from the Department of Infectology and 20 patients from the Internal Clinic. These departments represented the most dominant collection of material for this kind of diagnosis from the whole group of patients. The connection is proven precisely with the fact that patients from other inpatient departments, especially after operations, are transferred to the aftercare department, as well as the age limit in this department is shifted lower. The high incidence in the infectological clinic is due to the fact that diarrhea is a relatively frequent disease treated in this workplace. The internal clinic is the third in the order with the highest number of examinations to treat the group of patients where the polymorbidity, high age, immunocompromised state of the patient is high frequency.

Evaluation of Results by Diagnosis

Out of a total of 87 stool samples of patients screened for the presence of *Clostridium difficile*, 21 were received with the diagnosis of A09.0 Diarrhea and gastroenteritis of possibly infectious origin. This diagnosis is understandable, in most cases diarrhea patients are admitted to the infectological clinic. An equal number of 21 samples were received with a diagnosis related to the abdominal cavity, such as dyspepsia, ulcerative colitis, and irritable bowel syndrome. A lower incidence was the diagnosis of unspecified abdominal pain in 9 samples. Out of a total of 6 patients, the diagnosis related to septic disease developed. This number was also present in cardiovascular failure diagnoses.

Evaluation of Results with Respect to Other Risk Factors
Of the total number of toxin positive patients examined, up to 21 patients were partially immobile, 18 patients were fully immobile.

Of the total number of patients examined, 11 were assessed as polymorphic based on medical history data.

Abdominal surgery was performed in 8 patients out of the total. Immunocompromised condition was evaluated in 5 patients out of the total.

Of the total of 15 patients, oncological diagnosis such as prostate carcinoma was 3 patients, pancreatic cancer 2 patients, colon cancer 2 patients, NHL lymphoma 2 patients, breast cancer 1 patient, lung cancer 1 patient, esophageal cancer 1 patient and meningioma 1 patient.

Evaluation of Results with Respect to Antibiotic Therapy

Since the occurrence of *Clostridium difficile* toxins is related to the use of antibiotic therapy, we analyzed the type of antibiotic therapy in our study. Antibiotics from the cephalosporin group were present in 38 patients. This group of antibiotics is the largest. Antibiotics of this group were able to induce the formation of *Clostridium difficile* toxins after approximately 6-9 days of use. Another large group of antibiotics that occurred in patients in our test set and, after prolonged use, was able to induce CDI symptoms was the fluoroquinolone group. It occurred in 22 patients. Penicillin antibiotics have been reported in 20 patients in anamnestic data. Another large group was carbapenem antibiotics, which were used by 19 patients. In 10 patients, the use of aminoglycoside group antibiotics has been reported. Macrolides and imidazole derivatives occurred in 6 patients. In 5 patients of the whole group, antibiotics from the sulfonamide group were used for antibiotic therapy. The lowest incidence, only in 2 patients, were antibiotics from the group of glycopeptide antibiotics.

It should be noted that in our population most patients used a combination of multiple antibiotics. Often times in combination with metronidazole, which should act prophylactically against Clostridium difficile toxins, but in combination with another group of antibiotics, the effect for which it was administered did not occur.

Evaluation of Results Based on ATLAS

ATLAS - a predictive mortality scoring system in CDI patients that scores 5 critical risk factors (Age, Temperature, Leukocytosis, Albumin level, Systemic antibiotic administration during CD infection for more than 24 hours). Each of the above symptoms are assigned 0 to 2 points.

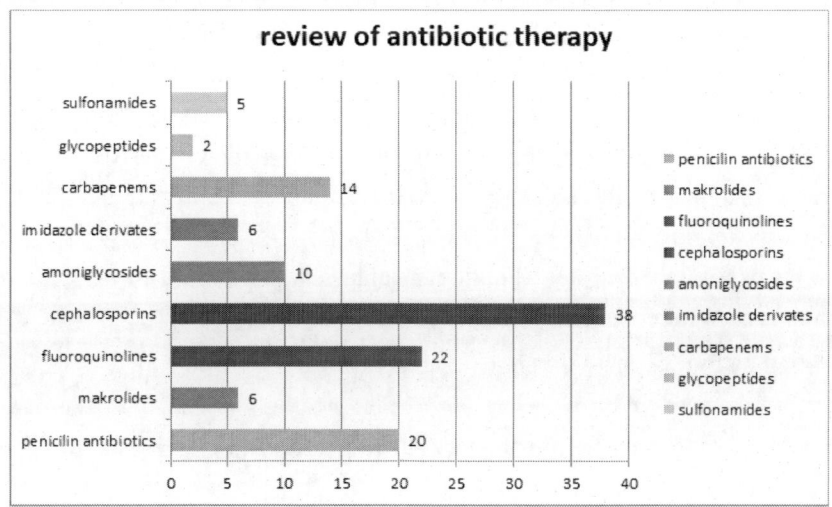

Figure 1. Review of antibiotic therapy.

Table 1. Atlas score

Parameter	0 points	1 point	2 point
Age	< 60 years	60 – 79 years	≥ 80 years
Temperature	≤ 37,5 °C	37,6 – 38,5 °C	≥ 38,6°C
Leukocytosis	< 16 000	16 000 – 25 000	> 25 000
Albumin level (g/L)	> 35	26 – 35	≤ 25
Systemic ATB therapy (≥ 1 day)	not	-	yes

Elevated temperature as a manifestation of infection was present from the entire group in 44 patients. For others, the elevated temperature was not recorded.

Monitoring of C-reactive protein values as a marker of inflammation was demonstrated in 84 patients from the entire set. It can be assessed that this indicator, together with the clinical condition of the patient (diarrhea when taking antibiotics), is very important in the diagnosis of CDI. Out of a total of 87 patients in 33 patients, elevated creatinine was reported. It cannot be verified that in other patients this value was negative as in some patients this indicator was not even investigated. Leukocytosis as one of the indicators of inflammation was present in 42 patients out of the total number of patients. The last parameter, the follow-up of elevated albumin levels, was found in only 4 patients after careful analysis in the patient's anamnestic records. Also, this data cannot be considered verified in our data as this parameter has not been investigated in all patients in our sample.

Out of a total of up to 10 patients, relapse was reported in our patient population. Where the most significant data is a relapse in a 75 year old female patient with 6 relapses.

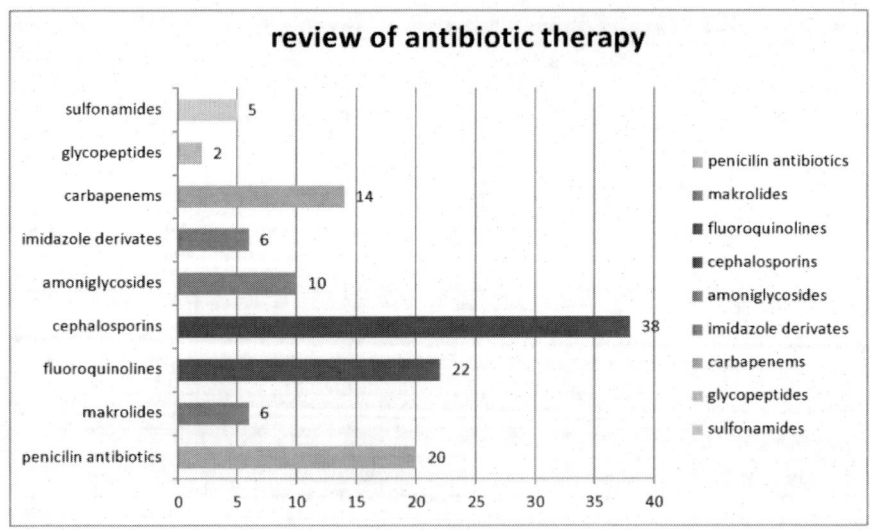

Figure 2. Monitoring of risk parameters monitoring.

CASUISTRY

75-year-old female patient with arterial hypertension, in the past appendectomy, repeatedly hospitalized in the internal ward of Trsena for diarrhea. In March 2017, the positivity of CD toxin, retreated with Vancomycin, Metronidazole. Progression complicated by acute myocardial infarction of the lower wall, solved by stent implantation. For diarrhea re-hospitalization in May 2017 in the internal ward of NsP Trstená, with a positive finding of CD Ag, toxin A + B. Vancomycin, Metronidazole indicated for treatment. Control microbiological examination after treatment with negat. found on CD Ag as well as toxin. In June 2017 again diarrhea with posit. CD Ag, toxin negat. Although the toxin was not detected, it was assumed that it was CDI. Indeed, the Clostridial toxin is very unstable if the patient's stool is not examined within two hours, the toxin decays very rapidly and a false negative result is obtained. Detection of the antigen is possible because the antigen does not disintegrate. Therefore, it is not possible to rely solely on detecting a toxin whose absence does not mean that the patient cannot have a Clostridial infection. Vancomycin, Metronidazole, Normix were indicated for treatment. For persistent chronic abdominal pain, watery stools about 7 times a day, with finding of palpable resistance in right hypogastria, weight loss about 15kg per half year, performed by internal department of NsP Trstena CT examination, sigmoscopy with finding of diverticulosis with sigmograph convection, . Examined by surgeon 28.06.2017, considered exploratory laparotomy, however, due to the time interval after overcoming IM, there was a high risk of perioperative complications. The patient was sent to the internal clinic of ÚVN SNP-Ružomberok - FN for the purpose of differentiating the condition. On admission, the patient reported chronic abdominal pain, in an objective finding the abdomen under the niveau of the chest, soft, palpable freely opaque in its entirety, palpalpation sensitive to the lower abdomen, Plenies, Rowsing, Blumberg negat. hatch diffuse tympanic, painless, peristalsis auscultantly present, irregular, without metal phenomena. X-ray of native abdomen does not show free air under diaphragms, levels in intestinal loops absent.

On June 1, 2017, the patient underwent pain in hypogastria, wind stop, 1x vomitus, the X-ray of the native abdomen without visible signs of free air under the diaphragms, numerous levels in the whole abdomen, diffuse gas filling in the intestine. A finding indicative of an ileous condition.

In the laboratory finding, mineral dysbalance, elevation of inflammatory parameters, administered infusion therapy, spasmo-analgesics. Consulted surgeon who recommended translation to surgical clinic. Introduced nasogastric tube and initiated intensive conservative treatment consisting of infusion therapy and correction of the internal environment. On July 08, 2017, the patient's condition is not improving, pain persists, in the X-ray of the native abdomen an illusory state with hypogastric levels persists, levels clearly formed, but the extent of GIT involvement to the same extent as 1.7.2017, without free gas under the diaphragms.

Explosive laparotomy with serous exudate colitis, abdominal cavity toilet, adhesiolysis, abdominal drainage, suture with ventrofil due to persistent illusion status. Due to repeated positive cultures for CD toxin ordained vancomycin at therapeutic dose + metronidazole + Fluconazole + Normix. Patient carotid, progressive weight loss of 20 kg, abdominal pain, repeated diarrhea persisted, woody plant deviates ascites fluid up to 1000 ml daily. Due to the positivity of the toxin CD consulted infectologist and patient transferred to the infectological clinic UVN SNP Ružomberok-FN on 11 July 2017. We used the ATLAS scoring system to assess the patient's health and risk of death. In our 75-year-old polymorphic patient, by assigning appropriate points to each symptom, the Median ATLAS score was 6. Due to the severe prognosis and persistence of CDI activity despite repeated treatment with vancomycin + metronidazole, we indicated fidaxomycin treatment that was refused by hospital management. Continued treatment with vancomycin + metronidazole at therapeutic dose and overall robotic treatment including protein saturation. Patient in improved condition August 2, 2017 released for home treatment. On August 7, 2017, recurrence of diarrhea with persistent CD antigen and toxin A, B persistence was recorded. Since the patient was exhausted from standard CDI treatment, due to age, polymorbidity was again indicated and approved by fidaxomycin. Treatment was started on August 15, 2017 with subsequent clinical improvement, and on August 25, 2017 in a stable state, released for home treatment. Fortunately, the patient did not die despite successful ATLAS score 6 due to successful treatment with fidaxomicin. In the following period, the relapse was no longer observed, a patient without dyspeptic complaints, overall well prospering.

DISCUSSION

Clostridial infections have an increasing trend in the world as well as in Slovakia. The increasing incidence is also supported by data provided by the Public Health Authority of the Slovak Republic. While in 2011 there were 136 cases of diseases reported in Slovakia, in 2017 their number increased to 2604 cases. However, the actual incidence of infections is higher. Many cases are not detected or underdiagnosed, there is a lack of standardization of data provided (Kreheľová, M., et al., 2018). Similarly, our research has shown an increased incidence of toxin positive samples. It also presents a problem in the treatment of the patient. A study conducted in hospitals in Mexico, as in our study, confirms that it is the antibiotics of the cephalosporin group that are the most common cause of postantibiotic diarrhea. In our study, 43.6 percent of patients used antibiotics of the cephalosporin group. In a study in Mexico, this figure was comparable to 47.0 percent (Hernaández - Giarcía, et al., 2015). Adult patients over the age of 65 are at increased risk for this type of infection and its more severe forms (Keller JM., et al., 2014). This has been confirmed in our analysis. In the study of the Canadian nosocomial infection surveillance program (CNISP), the authors evaluated the evolution of the epidemiological situation in Canadian hospitals during the post-epidemic period 2009-2015 also dominated by female sex, with a percentage of 49.7%. The group of patients over 65 years of age in this study was 65.8% (Katz, C.K, et al., 2018). In several articles we read about the possibility of laboratory diagnostics of *Clostridium difficile* by PCR method. We cannot realize this possibility in our laboratory. The diagnosis of the hyperviral R 02 compared to the 017 represents a more prevalent occurrence in Europe and North America (Imwattana, K., et al., 2019).

CONCLUSION

To determine the diagnosis of CDI, it is necessary to monitor the clinical condition of the patient, always consider the type of antibiotic therapy, take into account the risk factors in individual patients and ensure the spread of infection and adherence to the hygiene-epidemiological regimen to prevent nosocomial infection. The predictive scoring mortality system ATLAS can predict disease prognosis, predict recurrence and mortality. Based on our analysis, cephalosporin antibiotics represent a risk group. The prevention and prevention of infection is controlled and indicated by the use of antibiotics and targeted antibiotic therapy versus the use of broad spectrum antibiotics. In every patient with diarrhea occurring during antibiotic therapy, consideration should be given to screening for toxins of *Clostridium difficile*. Repeated microbiological diagnosis of *Clostridium difficile* toxins should not serve as a control of treatment efficacy for CDI, as the control of treatment efficacy is the improvement of the patient's clinical condition and the disappearance of CDI symptoms. An ideal therapy for CDI disease would be the obvious indication of fidaxomicin, which could be used automatically in patients who are at increased risk of complications based on ATLAS scores.

REFERENCES

Hernńdez-García R., Garza-González E., et.al. Application of the ATLAS score for evaluating the severity of *Clostridium difficile* infection in teaching hospital in Mexico, Braz. *Infect. Dis.*, 2015:19(4):399-402.
Guh AY, Mu Y, Baggs J, et al. Trends in incidence of long-term-care facility onset *Clostridium difficile* infections in 10 US geographic

locations during 2011-2015. *Am. J. Infect. Control* 2018. doi:10.1016/j.ajic.2017.11.026. [Epub ahead of print 9 Jan 2018].

Imwattna,K., Knight, D.R., et.al: Clostridium difficile ribotype 017 – characterization, evolution and epidemiology of the dominant strain in Asia, *Emerging Microbes & Infections* 2019, VOL. 8.

Jarčuška, P., Bátovský, M, Drdoňa, Ľ. et al. *Recommended procedure for the diagnosis and treatment of colitis caused by Clostridium difficile*, version 2.0, Via practica – Suplement 1, 2015, 12(S1).

Katz, CK, Golding, GR. The evolving epidemiology of Clostridium difficile infection in Canadian hospitals during a postepidemic period (2009–2015), *CMAJ*, 2018 Jun 25; 190(25): E758–E765.

Keller JM, Surawicz CM. *Clostridium difficile* infection in the elderly. *Clin. Geriatr. Med.* 2014;30:79-93.

Kreheľová, M., Sinajová, E.: Possibilities of laboratory diagnostics of infections caused by *Clostridium difficile*, *Newslab*, 2018, 9(2) : 86-90.

McDonald LC, Gerding DN, Johnson S, et al. Clinical practice guidelines for *Clostridium difficile* infection in adults and children: 2017 update by the Infectious Diseases Society of America (IDSA) and Society for Healthcare Epidemiology of America (SHEA). *Clin. Infect. Dis.* 2018 (published Online First: 2018/02/15).

Polák, P., Freibergerová, M., Husa, P. et al. Faecal bacteriotherapy in the treatment of recurrent colitis caused by *Clostridium difficile* at the Department of Infectious Diseases of the University Hospital Brno in 2010-2014 - prospective study. *Epidemiol. Mikrobiol. Imunol.*, 2015, 64:232-235.

Srivastava, A.; Talaue, M.; Liu, Shuang; Degen, David; Ebright, Richard Y; Sineva, Elena; Chakraborty, Anirban; Druzhinin, Sergey Y; Chatterjee, Sujoy; Mukhopadhyay, Jayanta; Ebright, Yon W; Zozula, Alex; Shen, Juan; Sengupta, Sonali; Niedfeldt, Rui Rong; Xin, Cai; Kaneko, Takushi; Irschik, Herbert; Jansen, Rolf; Donadio, Stefano; Connell, Nancy; Ebright, Richard H (2011). New target for inhibition of bacterial RNA polymerase: switch region. *Current Opinion in Microbiology*. 14 (5): 532–43.

In: Colitis: Causes, Diagnosis and Treatment   ISBN: 978-1-53616-631-6
Editor: Soren Garcia   © 2019 Nova Science Publishers, Inc.

Chapter 2

SULFATE SOURCE AND ITS ROLE IN THE DEVELOPMENT OF COLITIS

Ivan Kushkevych[*], *MSc, PhD, DrSc*
Department of Experimental Biology, Faculty of Science,
Masaryk University in Brno, Czech Republic

ABSTRACT

Inflammatory bowel disease (IBD), including ulcerative colitis (UC), is a complex multifactorial disease of unknown etiology. Intestinal sulfate-reducing bacteria (SRB), especially *Desuflovibrio* genus are often found in the intestines and feces of people and animals with IBD. One of the main roles in the development of UC among other factors can also be the species of this genus. These bacteria use sulfate as a terminal electron acceptor and organic compounds as an electron donor in their metabolisms. This fact leads us to the conclusion that sulfate present in the daily diet plays an important role in the development of bowel disease. Sulfate is present mainly in the following food commodities: i) some breads, soya flour, dried fruits, brassicas, and sausages; ii) as well as some beers, ciders, and wines. These data indicate that sulfate intake is highly dependent on diet. Literature data indicates that sulfate level

---

[*] Corresponding Author's E-mail: kushkevych@mail.muni.cz.

present in diet among people living in more developed countries consume over 16.6 mmole of sulfate per day. It should be noted the role of sulfite present in food since it can also be consumed by SRB. The complexity of sulfate metabolism can be overviewed by data that focuses on the intestinal environment containing different concentrations of hydrogen sulfide produced by SRB. According to the fact mentioned above, this chapter is dealing with issues concerning sulfate present in different food commodities and the intestinal environment affecting mainly SRB. These issues are explained by literature data indicating the role of sulfate in the intestines of animals, including humans. The data present in this chapter can be used to better explain of IBD and improve therapeutic strategies.

Keywords: inflammatory bowel disease, sulfate-reducing bacteria, *Desulfovibrio*, hydrogen sulfide

INTRODUCTION

Inflammatory bowel disease (IBD) represents a contemporary problem among a broader number of populations worldwide. According to statistical information it can be declared that IBD is a global disease in the 21st century. This fact can be especially labeled to the Europe and North America populations since the highest reported cases have been found there; ulcerative colitis 505 per 100,000 and 286 per 100,000 in Norway and in the USA, respectively. These numbers are probably more understandable when it is stated that over 1.5 million and 2 million people suffer from this disease in North America and Europe, respectively. The calculated prevalence in North America, Oceania, and many countries in Europe is 0.3%. The information that is indicating an increase of UC in newly industrialized countries in Africa, Asia, South America (including Brazil) should not be ignored. The information about the prevalence of IBD, including UC, has been unclear since recently. IBD is associated with morbidity, mortality, and substantial costs to the healthcare system [1, 2].

UC disease was first described by two English physicians, Wilks and Moxon, in 1875. Today UC in western countries is labeled as a complex and costly disease. Prevention is the best way of decreasing the incidence of IBD, including UC, especially because the prevalence is connected with environmental risks. The mortality rate among populations with UC is only slightly higher than in the general population [3].

UC is affecting mainly the working class of the population since the majority of diagnosed patients are between the ages of 30–40 years. Though certain literature data are indicating higher prevalence among people in the age group 60–69 years, same as among pediatric patients and adolescents. From these results it can be concluded that UC is probably an issue of high priority. The gender difference of UC is usually described in studies with a slight male predominance or significant differences between genders are not observed. There is a correlation between UC family history and UC prevalence, and genetic predisposition is usually connected with environmental risks. Contrary to many other diseases, nonsmokers have three times higher chance of developing UC. The following environmental conditions are connected with higher prevalence of UC: appendectomy (the data are not so clear that an appendectomy is a positive or negative factor influencing the development of UC), the presence of pathogenic microorganisms in the intestines, and malnutrition (usually associated with a poor quality of life) [4].

One of the main environmental risks for the development of IBD is the presence of sulfate in the daily diet and SRB in human intestines [5–10]. The sources of sulfate are: some breads, soya flour, dried fruits, brassicas, and sausages (high sulfate foods: > 10 μmol/g or 1 mg/g); some beers, ciders, and wines (high sulfate beverages: > 2.5 μmol/g or 0.25 mg/ml) [11, 12]. Sulfate content in the diet varies highly and can range from 2.1 mmol/day to 15.8 mmol/day [13]. The main percentage of sulfate from the diet is absorbed in the gut (more than 90% is used for assimilatory sulfate reduction, including synthesis of amino acids and proteins). The rest is used in the metabolic processes of SRB [13]. The absorption rate is highly dependent on each individual. SRB dissimilate sulfate as an electron acceptor to hydrogen sulfide in the dissimilatory sulfate reduction process. A correlation was found between the presence of SRB in the gut and the occurrence of IBD. This fact leads us to the main topic of our chapter since the sulfate presence in food and its absorption in the gut is related and will be discussed more in depth through subchapters. The chapter also contains a description for creating an experimental animal model of IBD based on sulfate-containing medium and injections of SRB suspension in the gastro-intestinal tract of rats. The main focus of the chapter is to describe the metabolic activity of SRB. Especially the species of *Desulfovibrio* genus because this genus is probably one of the main triggers that can be connected with the occurrence of IBD, including UC.

This chapter deals with issues concerning sulfate, SRB, and their influence on the development of IBD, including UC. The reviewed data present in this chapter describes the connection between the sulfate present in food, the presence of SRB in the intestines, and their overall influence on peoples' health. These newly found data will certainly improve our understanding of this aspect of IBD which can lead to better therapeutic strategies.

SULFATE CONTENT IN FOOD AND BEVERAGES

The sulfate in food is not comprehended as an important factor in human nutrition, especially because it is not considered as a source for the synthesis of amino acids. The fact is that sulfate is poorly absorbed. However, if the diet of a healthy person includes sulfate rich foods, the absorption is more than 16 mmol within 24 hours. Sulfate intake varies a lot among populations and can range from 2.1 mmol/day to 15.8 mmol/day [13]. In this case, absorbed sulfate can influence human requirements for methionine and cysteine [14]. The average person consumes about 20 mmol sulfate/day. One can do so by including these foods and said amounts into the diet: 200 g of bread (high sulfate bread), 100 g of sausages and 4 liters of beer. On the other hand, sulfate present in the diet, if not absorbed in the small bowel, starts to be a potential substrate for sulfate-reducing bacteria found in colonic lumen [13]. Sulfate-reducing bacteria are anaerobes that are able to dissimilate sulfate to hydrogen sulfide; hydrogen sulfide represents a toxic compound for the colonic mucosa [5, 15-18]. The daily intake of sulfate among the USA population is 453 mg [19]. Other literature data are indicating that the Western diet contains 1.6 mmol of sulfate/day and the African diet 2.7 mmol of sulfate/day [13].

According to Florin the highest sulfate concentrations were found in dried apple (> 5 mg/g). Dried fruits are often sulfured by sulfur dioxide (E_{220}), sulfite (E_{221}), and disulfite (E_{227}). This practice leads to the occurrence of higher sulfate amounts in food. The amount of sulfur dioxide – sulfites (E_{220}–E_{228}) – allowed to be added to aromatized wines, aromatized wine-base drinks, and aromatized wine-product cocktails is 10 mg/kg or 10 mg/l [20]. According to European Regulation Law 1169/2011, prepacked food should be labeled to contain sulfite if their level exceeds 10 mg/l (expressed as SO_2). The role of SO_2 as a sulfate source, influence of metabolic processes, and use by intestinal sulfate-reducing bacteria has been insufficiently studied.

The European Food Safety Authority (EFSA) gave their scientific opinion about the following food additives that can be a source of sulfur in food: sulfur dioxide (E_{220}), sodium sulfite (E_{221}), sodium bisulfite (E_{222}), sodium metabisulfite (E_{223}), potassium metabisulfite (E_{224}), calcium sulfite (E_{226}), calcium bisulfite (E_{227}), and potassium bisulfite (E_{228}). The scientific opinion stressed that acceptable daily intake (ADI) (for all population groups) of SO_2 is 0.7 mg of SO_2 equivalent/kg of body weight per day, though it is also mentioned that this amount probably will be updated in the future with more precise studies, such studies need 5 years for completion (EFSA, 2016) [21].

It is important to stress that these results are from 1993 and since that time the results for the amount of sulfate present in food have not been updated. It is considered that traditionally the most important sources of sulfate in the diet are beer, bread, sausages, and cabbage. The food in which sulfate occurs naturally are grapes, nuts, coconut milk, avocado, crustacea, and shellfish. These food commodities are important for the sulfate requirements of sulfate conjugation, same for molecules like chondroitin sulfate. Sulfate intake has a positive effect on the protein sparing effect since proteins in certain diets (for an example, among some African populations) are very scarce. Sulfate conjugation is an important pathway in the processes of detoxification and excretion of many drugs and xenobiotics. It means that sulfate included in the diet is accelerating drug metabolism. One study found [13] that a diet rich in brassica (150 g sprouts and 100 g cabbage) had stimulating effects on phenolic drug metabolism. These high sulfate food commodities are not labeled though consumers can be informed about the possible higher quantity of sulfate intake, caused by the consumption of these kind of foods. Contrarily, the presence and amount of sulfite is labeled on the packaging of beverages, sausages, jams and dried fruits.

It was already mentioned the main food commodities of sulfate source. It should be also emphasized that there is high variation between results and it does not mean that certain food commodities would always represent high sulfate source due to different amounts present in food. For an example, one cola brand can have 8 times higher sulfate content than other cola brand. The same trend was also found within the same manufacturer. The staple foods are a type of food that can easily affect a broader number of people, since it consumed in high quantities among the majority of the population. Out of staple food products, besides bread, it was also found that potatoes are a source for a higher exposure of sulfate. The source of sulfate is sulfuring of soya flour, nuts, grape and tomato juice.

Bread is a source of sulfate due to the addition of ferrous sulfate, calcium sulfate, ammonium sulfate, sulfur dioxide, or sodium disulfite. Consequently, individual ingredients of bread can be neglected sources of sulfate, but due to the addition additives during bread production it starts to be a food with high sulfate content (Table 1).

Table 1. The sulfate content in some food types (data are calculated from the research of Florin et al. 1991)

Sulfate due to processing		Natural occurring sulfate	
Type of foods	Sulfate (μmole/gram)	Type of foods	Sulfate (μmole/gram)
Bread	12 ± 3.60	Grapes	1.9 ± 0.70
Beer	1.43 ± 1.11	Nuts	6.03 ± 2.89
Dried fruits	21.5 ± 2.18	Coconut milk	5 ± 1.6
Sausages	6 ± 5.65	Avocado	5.2 ± 0.28

Permitted additives added during bread manufacturing are ferrous, calcium, and ammonium sulfate [22]. In homemade bread, sulfate content is usually relatively low. This kind of food manipulation during processing can also lead to a switch between low and high sulfate source in other food commodities. This fact can be added to the observation that mainly foods high in sulfate are processed foods and sulfate was added to them during their production. The presence of glucosinolate compounds in food such as the brassica vegetable can also lead to higher sulfate concentrations due to the chance that glucosinolates can easily cleave to sulfate under heat treatment or in mild acid environment. The study also found positive correlations ($p < 0.05$) between glucosinolate amount and sulfate in vegetables [23, 24]. Vegetables, such as cabbage, are naturally rich in sulfate due to glucosinolate content. Sulfite or disulfite is added to fruit and vegetables as a preservative during their processing. These preservative compounds are also the source of sulfate since some sulfite can oxidize to sulfate during the storage period or during heat treatment of these products [24].

Drinking water is also a source of sulfate due to the following naturally occurring minerals: barite ($BaSO_4$), epsomite ($MgSO_4 \times 7H_2O$), and gypsum ($CaSO_4 \times 2H_2O$). Sulfate has been observed to be present in drinking water in the shape of sodium sulfate and calcium sulfate in concentrations up to 100 mg/liter.

Also, and unusual fact is that people begin to dislike the taste of water with a sulfate concentration of 850 mg/ml, though sensory properties of distilled water were improved when sulfate ranged from 90 to 270 mg/ml [25]. Ferrous sulfate is also added to drinking water during processing [13].

The sulfate concentrations in food are growing due to the presence of sulfate in the production of fertilizers, chemical, dyes, paper, glass, soaps, fungicides, insecticides, emetics and astringents, during mining, wood pulp, metal and plating industries, leather processing, in sewage treatment, in drinking water treatment and the chemicals used for the controlling of algae [26, 27].

Beer is considered high in sulfate, but correlations were not found between the presence of sulfite and sulfate concentrations [11]. Few amounts of sulfate in beer can be formed during fermentation (sulfite is transformed to sulfate) and also due to sulfuring of hops. A higher amount of sulfate in beer can be found in bitter beers where calcium sulfate is added to reduce the pH of the mash [12]. Certain studies have been indicating that beer consumption can lead to a higher prevalence of colorectal cancer. Florin et al. (1991) stated that beer consumption leads to a more sulfate rich diet. It serves SRB production of hydrogen sulfide which can affect the prevalence of colorectal cancer [13, 28, 29]. The diversity of sulfate sources can be also overviewed by the fact that sulfate contents are found in rain and can represent a source of sulfate (in Canada: 1.0 to 3.8 mg/l) [30]. Sulfide produced by SRB in the colon can lead to cancer, but a direct connection cannot be made between sulfide in the colon and cancer prevalence, it can only cause leakage of mucosal epithelium to carcinogens in feces [11, 12].

The sulfate content in food has multiple sources. Some sulfate occurs naturally in certain food types, but some sulfate is added externally to food in the processing. Compounds containing sulfate are starting to be studied more extensively since recently completed studies are not giving a clear picture about the role of sulfate included in the diet. It is certain that future studies will evaluate more precisely the adequate amount of sulfate that is recommended in the daily diet. SRB will also stay connected with sulfate consumption studies since their activities correlate with the use/consumption/absorption of sulfate from food in human metabolism.

Thus, sulfate content in food and beverages depends on their type. Sufficient amounts of sulfate can be found in the food (bread, rice, soya, etc.), fresh vegetables (broccoli, brussels sprouts, avocado, potato, spinach, etc.), fresh fruits (coconut, kiwi, plum, etc.), beverages (tomato juice, coffee, beer, etc.) and also in drinking water. These amounts depend on if the food was processed or not, and if the food was cooked or uncooked. Sulfate in cooked food is mainly in the free anionic form. On the other hand, sulfate from intestinal secretions is esterified with glycoproteins (mainly mucin) and to a lesser extent with steroids and glycolipids. The source of sulfate in the diet of different populations may vary and depends on the type of food consumed.

SULFATE ABSORPTION IN THE GUT

Colonic pathophysiology can be affected by dietary sulfate since it is influencing sulfate-reducing bacteria in the bowel [5, 29, 31]. These bacteria are transforming sulfate into hydrogen sulfide that is potentially toxic for the bowel environment [15, 18, 28]. On the other hand, it is still not clearly described and evaluated the amount of sulfate reaching bowel. A study, conducted with six healthy ileostomists and three healthy non ileostomists, individuals were fed a diet containing 1.6 mmol/day to 16.6 mmol/day of sulfate [13]. The results found a maximum sulfate absorption of 5 mmol/day to 16 mmol/day in ileostomists and normal individuals, respectively. Up to 9 mmol/day of sulfate reached the colon. The excretion of sulfate in feces was less than 0.5 mmol/day. The study showed that sulfate content in the colon, where it can be used by sulfate-reducing bacteria, highly influences and is a positively correlated with dietary sulfate. The absorption of sulfate in the upper gastrointestinal tract was almost similar in both groups (healthy normal and health ileostomists individuals). It was also found that favorable bound sulfate was found only in normal individuals without ileostomy. Bound sulfate is formed out of aromatic amino acids degradation. The excretion of bound sulfate in the study [13] was 0.16 mmol/day, sulfate 0.26 mmol/day, and free faecal sulfate 0.10 mmol/day. The amount of dietary sulfate does not increase significantly ($p < 0.05$) its feces excretion. On the other hand, urinary sulfate excretion has a positive sign correlation ($p < 0.05$) with dietary sulfate [13].

The maximum absorption of sulfate was reached in the study where subjects excreted 52 mmol of sulfate per day by urine (they were fed by 380 mmol of sulfate during four hours). It was found that excessive amounts of sulfate possess laxative properties. Lower amounts of sulfate given to volunteers (60 mmol of sulfate in three divided doses during 24 hours) gave results that 62% of the sulfate was excreted during three days [32]. The main source of sulfate is still the oxidation of sulfur containing amino acids (methionine and cysteine); calculated to be around 20 mmol/day.

Summarized sulfate in the colon has the following pathway (Figure 1):

- It is consumed by sulfate-reducing bacteria (as an electron acceptor), and transformed into hydrogen sulfide.
- It is consumed by other intestinal bacteria (*Clostridium, Escherichia, Klebsiela*...) capable of consuming sulfate and producing hydrogen sulfide.
- Part of hydrogen sulfide in the colon is excreted as a gas.
- Part of hydrogen sulfide is absorbed in the colon and reoxidized into sulfate.

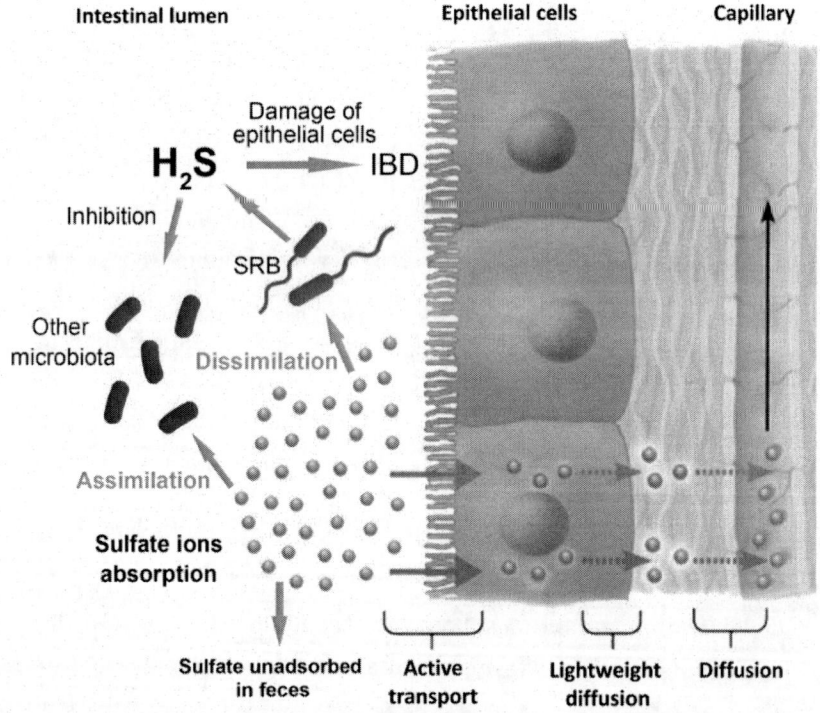

Figure 1. The scheme of sulfate absorption in the gut.

The produced hydrogen sulfide is fortunately readily absorbed if not included in chemical or enzymatic reactions. It was estimated that fecal bacteria (without sulfate-reducing bacteria) needs only maximum

2 mmol/day of sulfur. This amount is easily achieved by cysteine and methionine degradation. When the zero sulfate diet was applied, urinary excretion of sulfate was 19.4 mmol/day [13].

Net endogenous sulfate secretion by the human upper gastrointestinal tract was estimated to be from 0.96 mmol/day to 2.6 mmol/day. Sulfate is mainly presented in mucin, but can be also bounded to esters of steroids, glycoproteins, phenols, chondroitin and glycolipids. The amount of sulfate in the small intestinal and gastric mucin is much lower than in colonic mucin. The incorporation of blood sulfate into mucin is rapid [33].

Bounded sulfate is lost to ileostomy fluid. When sulfate intakes are at the highest levels, a significant increase was noticed in ileal bound sulfate: 0.06 mmol/mmol ingested sulfate. This can be explained by the increased sulfation of secreted substances and increased endogenous secretion. Certainly there is the possibility of systematic error in the sulfate measurement [13]. Total sulfate content/pool in the colon depends almost entirely on endogenous sulfate. Diet (though it is considered that sulfate is poorly absorbed by human gastrointestinal tract) and intestinal absorption are the main factors affecting the amount of sulfate present in the colon [11, 12]. The amount of the sulfate present in the colon affects SRB and their sulfide production [34, 35].

Sulfate in the human body can have also osmotic laxative properties. The source of sulfate found in urine can be from the oxidation of amino acids containing sulfur. Though studies are showing that a certain amount of sulfate is absorbed from diet by the upper gastrointestinal tract and can be excreted in urine during 24 hours after intake [12, 13]. Since there is little sulfatase activity in the mucosa, it can be stated that most likely the free sulfate in ileal effluent is of dietary origin [13].

Thus, sulfate absorption in the gut depends on many factors and can vary. It may be genetically determined in each individual. The sulfate level in the intestine can also depend on the number of SRB and their dissimilatory sulfate reduction process.

PROCESS OF SULFATE REDUCTION

The process of sulfate reduction can be divided into two pathways: "dissimilatory sulfate reduction" and "assimilatory sulfate reduction" [5,14]. The dissimilatory sulfate reduction is a complex and multistage process, in which SRB consume sulfate as terminal electron acceptor and reduce it to hydrogen sulfide [15]. The assimilatory sulfate reduction is characteristic of all living organisms. In this case, the sulfate is reduced to hydrogen sulfide, which is further involved in metabolism, in particular in the synthesis of sulfur-containing organic compounds such as a cysteine or methionine [36]. The scheme of both processes is presented in Figure 2.

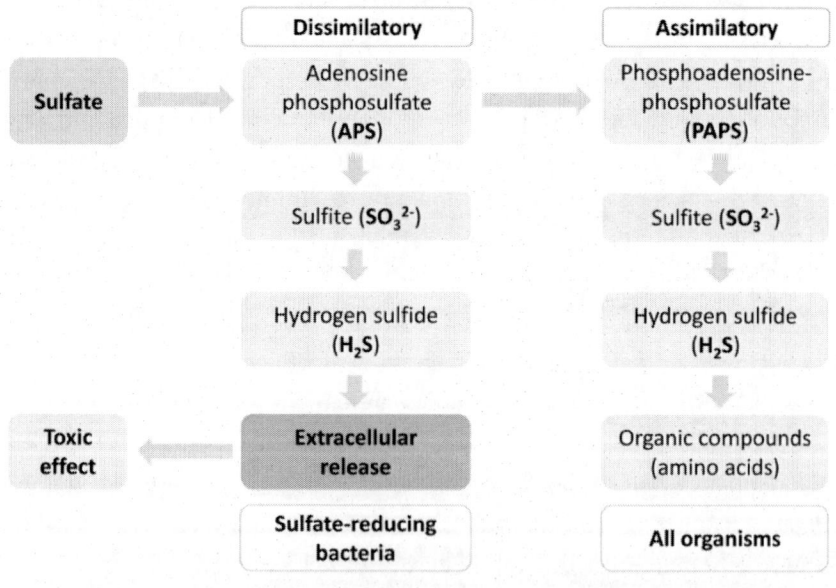

Figure 2. The scheme of comparing of dissimilatory and assimilatory sulfate reduction.

As was noted above, the presence of sulfate in the intestine does not only depend on the absorption of gut properties, but also on the activity of sulfate-reducing bacteria that can dissimilate it to toxic hydrogen sulfide. So, the process of dissimillatory sulfate reduction of in this chapter is characterized in more detail.

The enzymes of SRB involved in the process of dissimilatory sulfate reduction are localized as in the cytoplasm and also in the periplasm. At the beginning stages of sulfate reduction, sulfate is absorbed in a bacterial cell [8]; sulfate can be transported into the cells simultaneously with protons. Some halophilic SRB species can absorb sulfate together with the flow of sodium ions [14]. Dissimilatory sulfate reduction can be divided into following stages (see Figure 2).

Sulfate transported into bacterial cells is activated by the enzyme ATP sulfurylase (EC 2.7.7.4), which transfers sulfate to adenosine monophosphate moiety of ATP with the formation of adenosine 5'-phosphosulfate (APS) and pyrophosphate (PP_i) [37]. The reaction is also reversible, and therefore, ATP can be formed from APS and PP_i [38, 39]. ATP sulfurylase catalyzes the following reaction (Figure 3):

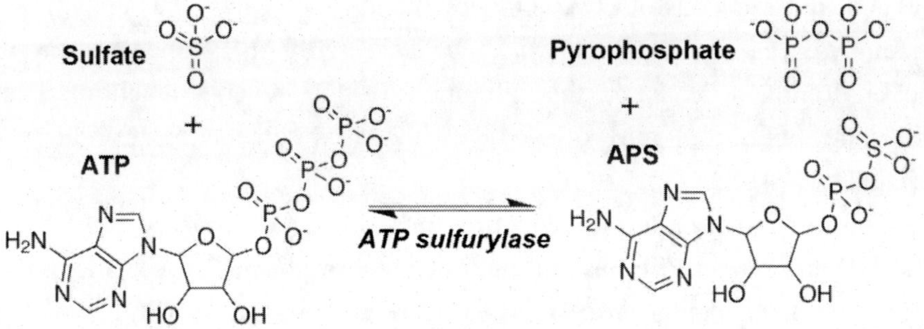

Figure 3. The reaction of sulfate and ATP catalyzed by ATP sulfurylase (modified from Ravilious et al. 2013) [40].

ATP sulfurylase is coded by the *sat* gene. This enzyme found in the cells of many different organisms differs by molecular weight, and mono-, di-, tetra- or hexameric structure. Most ATP sulfurylases consist of identical subunits containing cobalt and zinc ions [5, 14]. ATP sulfurylases of *Desulfovibrio desulfuricans* and *D. gigas* are homotrimers with molecular weights of 141 and 147 kDa, respectively. The *Desulfovibrio* genus contains cytoplasmic pyrophosphatase (EC 3.6.1.1) which catalyzes the cleavage of pyrophosphate into two phosphate ions [38]. In the process of pyrophosphate hydrolysis, energy is released in the form of a transmembrane proton potential [14].

Sulfate activation leads to an increase of redox potential (E^0) from -516 mV to -60 mV [5,14]. An increase of E^0 provides the reduction of APS, which serves as an electron acceptor. The species of the *Desulfovibrio* genus contains cytoplasmic APS reductase (adenylyl-sulfate reductase, EC 1.8.99.2) that promotes the reduction of APS to sulfite or bisulfite and AMP [41,42,43] by the following reaction:

$$APS \xrightarrow{APS\ reductase} SO_3^{2-} + AMP$$

APS reductase is a nonheme iron-sulfur containing flavoprotein with a molecular weight of 95 kDa, which consists of α- and β-subunits. The first (α) subunit contains a molecule of flavin adenine dinucleotide and the second (β) contains two [4Fe–4S]-centers [14,41,42]. APS reductase was isolated from the cells of *D. desulfuricans* and *D. vulgaris*. This enzyme is coded by two genes: *aprA* and *aprB*. An increase of AMP concentration in the environment leads to the inhibition of the reverse reaction. The concentration of 1.8 mM of AMP or more causes the reaction to be terminated [14].

The dissimilatory sulfate reduction to H_2S in SRB occurs also through the formation of sulfite as an intermediate product [5]. So, the next important stage in this process is sulfite reduction. Sulfite (SO_3^{2-}) is the product of APS reduction and more reactive than sulfate. Reduction of SO_3^{2-} to S^{2-} is catalysed by dissimilatory sulfite reductase (EC 1.8.99.1), which can be coded by three genes (*dsvA, dvsB, dsvC*). This enzyme is usually composed of two α- and β-subunits (α2β2) [44,45]. However, the bacteria *D. vulgaris* and *D. desulfuricans* Essex contain a third subunit (γ). Dissimilatory sulfite reductase in these microorganisms is a hexamer (α2β2γ2) [14]. Active centers of sulfite reductases have two metal ion cofactors, siroheme, and [FeS]-cluster [46]. They are involved in the transport of electrons. Six electrons are transported in the reduction of sulfite to hydrogen sulfide [47,48,49]. SRB have the following types of dissimilatory sulfite reductases: (1) Desulfoviridine, (2) Desulforubidine, (3) Desulfofuscidine, and (4) Protein P_{582} [5,49].

Bisulfite is one form of sulfite. Some scientists believe that actual substrate in the process of dissimilatory sulfite reduction is bisulfite rather than sulfite [14]. That is why sulfite reductase is often also called bisulfite reductase [49].

Sulfite reductase plays an important role in the process of assimilation of sulfur. The enzyme promotes the formation of sulfide for synthesis of sulfur-containing amino acids including methionine and cysteine. This enzyme is found in the cells of *Desulfovibrio* genus as well as in many other SRB [5, 50].

Sulfide is formed after repeated reduction by two electrons and the subsequent protonation of oxygen atoms, which are then gradually removed from the atoms of sulfur. Bisulfite reduction through three two-electron steps can be faster than only one step using six electrons [14]. If SRB are grown in the presence of bisulfite or thiosulfate, it is possible that they might not use sulfate as the primary electron acceptor [51].

Summing up the dissimilatory sulfate reduction process, it should be noted that hydrogen sulfide formed from sulfite is released into the intestinal lumen. Therefore, the concentration of hydrogen sulfide in the intestinal lumen and its detection in the feces depends on the intensity of sulfate reduction and, respectively, the SRB number in the intestine. In the assimilatory sulfate reduction process, APS is converted to phosphoadenosine phosphosulfate by the enzyme APS kinase. This process is similar to the dissimilatory sulfate reduction, but in this case hydrogen sulfide is used in anabolism and converted to cesteine by O-acetylserine-(thiol)-lyase A/B [52]. The genes coding this enzyme are *CysK* and *CysM* [53].

The dissimilatory sulfate reduction and also assimilatory sulfate reduction processes require exogenous electron donors [5, 14]. Such the universal donor for SRB is molecular hydrogen [5]. Oxidation of molecular hydrogen can occur in the periplasm and also in the cytoplasm by the enzyme called hydrogenases. Hydrogenases are the enzymes that catalyze the reversible redox reaction in the presence of hydrogen. They play an important role in anaerobic respiration [54]. Hydrogen oxidation is caused by the reduction of the terminal electron acceptor (oxygen, nitrate, sulfate, carbon (IV) oxide, and fumarate) [14]. Reduction of H_2 is important for transforming pyruvate. Some molecules and proteins (ferredoxin, cytochrome c_3 and cytochrome c_6) can be physiological donors or acceptors of electrons for hydrogenases. Hydrogenases are involved in the absorption and formation of molecular hydrogen. This process occurs through the reaction [49]:

$$H_2 \rightleftharpoons H^+ + H^- \rightleftharpoons 2H^+ + 2\bar{e}$$

Four types of periplasmic hydrogenases are known: [NiFe], [FeFe], [NiFeSe] and [Fe]. The metal ions play an important role in the functioning of the active centers of all hydrogenases. *D. vulgaris* contains four hydrogenases, including three [NiFe]-hydrogenases (EC 1.12.99.6) and one [FeFe]-hydrogenase (EC 1.12.7.2) [14, 55]. These four types of hydrogenases can completely functionally change each other, especially when bacteria growing in the medium with higher concentrations of H_2 [56]. In the cytoplasm, the process of molecular hydrogen oxidation is not achieved only by cytoplasmic hydrogenase, but also FeS proteins are involved [5]. SRB *D. vulgaris* contains two membrane complexes of hydrogenase, EchABCDEF and CooMKLXUHF, which are interrelated [57, 58]. They catalyze the reduction of ferredoxins in the presence of H_2 or protons to H_2 through ferredoxin reduction. Both of these reductions cause the formation of a proton electrochemical potential [55]. Thus, cytoplasmic hydrogenases catalyze not only H_2 oxidation, but also the reduction of ferredoxin [59]. It should be noted, that the molecular hydrogen in the intestine can be produced by clostridia [60] and used by SRB as an electron donor [61, 62]. However, the SRB can compete for hydrogen with methanogenic microorganisms that may inhibit the process of methanogenesis [63, 64].

Other alternative electron donors for SRB are organic compounds which may also be used as carbon and an energy source [5]. In the large intestine, the most common electron donors for SRB, except for molecular hydrogen, are lactate (produced by lactic acid bacteria), acetate, propionate, amino acids, short chain fatty acids, succinate, ethanol, and many others. These can be formed in the fermentation process [14, 34]. The scheme of oxidation of electron donor in the process of dissimilatory sulfate reduction is presented in Figure 4.

The oxidation of organic compounds as an electron donor can be done completely with the formation of CO_2 or incompletely with acetate formation [5]. For example, lactate can be oxidized incompletely to acetate by the *Desulfovibrio* or *Desulfomicrobium* species. Other SRB species can consume acetate as an electron donor and a carbon source. In this case, acetate is oxidized to CO_2. The species of *Desulfobulbus propionicus* can use propionate, which is later oxidized to acetate and CO_2 [49, 65].

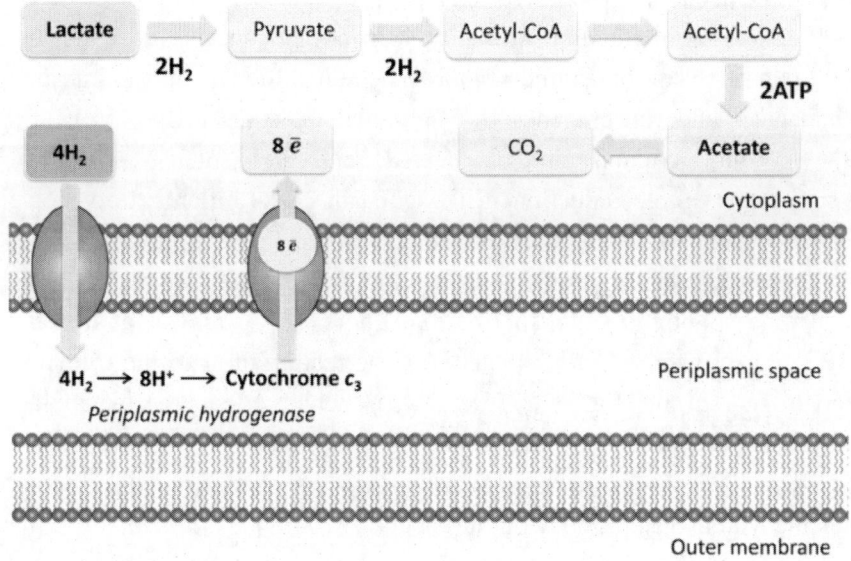

Figure 4. The scheme of electron donor oxidation in the process of dissimilatory sulfate reduction.

Thus, sulfate reduction to hydrogen sulfide occurs through intermediates (APS and SO_3^{2-}), which play the role of electron acceptors. These intermediates are not released by SRB into the intestinal lumen. The main electron donors in the intestine are H_2, lactate, acetate, propionate, and other organic compounds.

SULFATE-REDUCING BACTERIA AND BOWEL DISEASE

W. E. Moore was the first to isolate intestinal SRB from the feces in 1976 [66]. This culture was identified as *Desulfomonas pigra* and subsequently reclassified to *Desulfovibrio piger* [67]. Later, the following genera belonging to the intestinal microbiota of humans and animals were isolated: *Desulfovibrio*, *Desulfomicrobium*, *Desulfobulbus*, *Desulfobacter*, *Desulfomonas*, and *Desulfotomaculum* [14, 34, 65, 68, 69]. As was already noted in the previous subchapter, the presence of sulfate, molecular hydrogen, and lactate in the human intestine contributes to their intensive growth and accumulation of hydrogen sulfide.

Production of hydrogen sulfide by SRB in high concentrations can lead to a toxic effect on other microbiota, and their inhibition in the intestine, mutagenesis and cancer genesis of epithelial intestinal cells [15, 17, 28, 29]. So, the increased number of SRB and their intense process of dissimilatory sulfate reduction in the gut can cause inflammatory bowel diseases of humans and animals [16, 17, 34].

These bacteria are often found in persons with rheumatic diseases and ankylosing spondylitis, etc. [5, 14, 28]. There is also an assumption that SRB can cause some forms of cancer in the rectum through the formation of hydrogen sulfide (Figure 5) [28, 29, 31], which affects the metabolism of intestinal cells and gives rise to various IBD [5, 29].

SRB, *Desulfovibrio*, and *Desulfomonas* genera from the human intestine were isolated by J. Loubinoux et al. (2002) [71]. It is believed that SRB are not pathogenic in humans and animals [5, 14]. However, they can cause various diseases together with other infections [34]. The species of *Desulfovibrio* genus, including *D. fairfieldensis*, are the most often isolated among all SRB during the disease [72, 73]. The species of this genus play, obviously, a bigger role in pathogenesis than other species of SRB. Bacteria *D. fairfieldensis* were isolated during mono- and polymicrobial infections of the gastrointestinal tract [74]. In total, 12 of 100 samples of purulent abdominal, and pleural cavities contained human *D. piger*, *D. fairfieldensis*, or *D. desulfuricans* [73].

SRB *D. desulfuricans* causing bacteremia was isolated from the bleeding microvilli of the colon [74]. This research shows that the main way SRB penetrate the blood vessels is through the damaged intestinal microvilli and then the bacteria cause an infection. SRB is also detected in the oral cavity [72, 75]. Similarly to some methanogens, they can cause the development of other diseases, including cholecystitis, abscesses of the brain and abdomen, ulcerative enterocolitis, cancer, etc. [5, 6, 14]. The species of *Desulfovibrio* genus also caused bloody diarrhea, weight loss, anorexia, epithelial hyperplasia, abscesses, and inflammatory infiltrates in animals and humans [5, 29, 31, 34, 76].

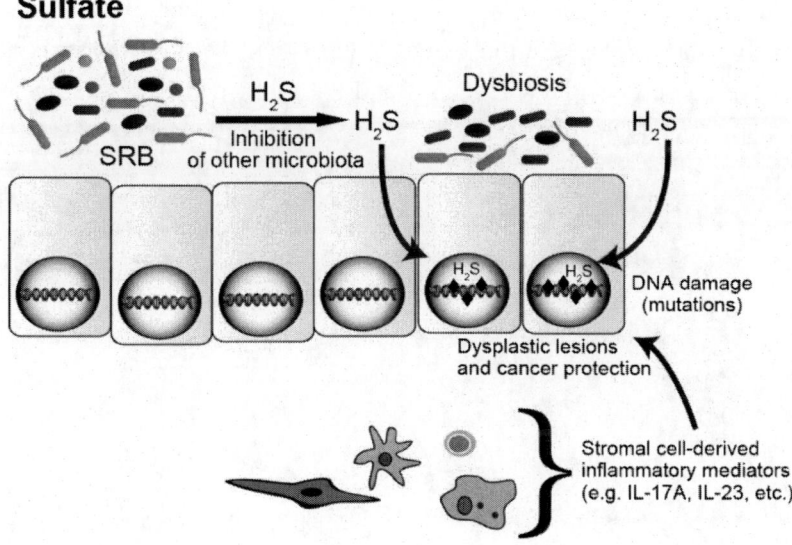

Figure 5. Possible cancer rectum development through DNA damage by H_2S (the scheme is modified from Jobin, 2013) [70].

An increased number of SRB was found in feces of people with ulcerative colitis compared with healthy individuals [34]. The injection of these bacteria in hamster intestine caused an infection that is clinically similar to human colitis [77]. The bacteria of this genus caused a pyogenic liver abscess [78] and bacteremia [79] (Figure 6).

Prevalence of SRB varies in different people. These microorganisms were found in the feces of 70% of healthy people in the United Kingdom and only in 15% of the inhabitants of Africa. SRB number observed in the stool of 143 healthy people ranged from 10^2 to 10^{11} cells/g of feces [34]. Another study with 87 healthy people found that the number of SRB ranged from 10^7 to 10^{11} cells/g of feces. It differs among residents of different areas [34, 35]. As already mentioned, the species of the *Desulfovibrio* genus were always dominant among SRB in the gut. They account for 67–91% of total SRB numbers. Significantly fewer bacteria are found from *Desulfobacter* (9–16%), *Desulfobulbus* (5–8%), and *Desulfotomaculum* (2%) genera [5, 34]. SRB producing the largest number of hydrogen sulfide were isolated from feces of the human distal colon. It is probably due to the reaction of the environment because the proximal part of the colon is acidic (pH < 5.5) and the distal part is neutral [5, 14, 34, 35].

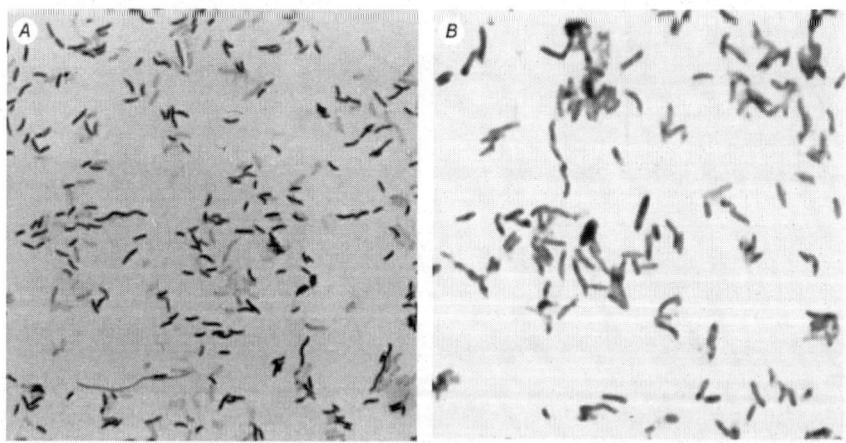

Figure 6. Bacteria *Desulfovibrio* genus isolated from different objects
(light microscopy, × 1,000): (*A*) isolates caused a pyogenic liver abscess (photo by Tee et al. 1996) [78], (*B*) isolates caused bacteremia (photo by McDougall et al. 1996) [79].

It has been found that SRB are available not only in the feces, but they also colonize the intestinal mucosa and form biofilm with other bacteria (e.g., *Bacteroides*, *Pseudomonas*, or *Clostridium*, etc.) [80–83]. As a result, the samples from men and women acquired by the rectal biopsy contain from 10^6 to 10^7 CFU/g of biopsy [84]. In the mucosa of some people, the number of *Desulfovibrio* species is changed by several orders during the period of 12 months. It probably is dependent on the nutrition of these individuals. SRB colonize the intestines of humans right from the beginning of their lives [84]. The presence of the *Desulfovibrio* genus was detected in the feces of infants under the age of six months. The number of *Desulfovibrio* species in these children, which were breast-fed or bottle-fed, was 3.7×10^3 and 4.5×10^4 cells/g of feces, respectively [14, 34].

Bacteria on the surface of the colon mucosa are in close relationship with the human body [5]. They interact with the cells of the immune and neuroendocrine systems more closely than microorganisms in the intestine lumen [81, 82, 83]. It is believed that the species composition and the number of SRB on the surface of the intestinal mucosa differ from microorganisms in its lumen [80]. The presence of sulfate ions promotes the growth of intestinal SRB, which use molecular hydrogen and compete with methanogenic microorganisms for this universal electron donor [35].

As already mentioned in the previous subchapter, the SRB can oxidize a range of readily available organic compounds in the colon (short chain fatty acids, hydrogen, succinate, lactate, ethanol, and pyruvate) and are likely to be growth limited not by substrate, but by the availability of the terminal electron acceptor, which is sulfate [5]. Large numbers of SRB were detected in the colon, especially in people who did not excrete methane in their breath [85]. It is suggested that these microorganisms might outgrow methanogenic bacteria when there is an adequate supply of sulfate [35]. The amount of sulfate available in the colon and the relative contributions of the diet and endogenous secretions is important to know, to understand more fully its role in determining SRB activity [13].

It is believed that the sulfate is poorly absorbed by the human gastrointestinal tract [13]. So, based on this property, it can be used as an osmotic laxative, and as a non-absorbable anion in absorption studies [12, 13]. Glycoproteins (mainly mucin), and to a lesser extent steroids and glycolipids, contain sulfated residuals, which can also be used as a source of sulfate for SRB. The free sulfate in ileal effluent is likely to be of dietary origin, whereas bound sulfate is largely endogenous [86]. It is assumed that sulfate losses in ileal effluent are the same as the sulfate, which reaches the caecum in the intact gut [13]. Probably, the contribution of endogenous sulfate to the total colonic sulfate pool is small. However, the amount of sulfate released from the colonic mucin can also be an important factor for the intestinal SRB activity and their production of hydrogen sulfide [5]. Moreover, it is known that colonic mucin is more highly sulfated than small intestinal and gastric mucin [87]. Consequently, the metabolism and activity of mucin-degrading colonic bacteria may also be no less an important factor for SRB growth. For example, clostridia, on one hand, can cleave the complex organic compounds such as mucin and, on the other hand, produce molecular hydrogen which SRB can use as an electron donor. Therefore, it is very important to study such relationships of SRB with clostridia and other intestinal bacteria in not only the bowel lumen, but also in the composition of biofilms.

Thus, the etiological role of SRB in the development of diseases is obvious. The presence of free sulfate in the intestine activates the growth of SRB and, accordingly, their production of hydrogen sulfide. High concentrations of this final metabolite of SRB can have both mutagenic and carcinogenic effects. The species of *Desulfovibrio* genus are the most often isolated among all SRB during various diseases. That is why SRB in intestinal microbial composition plays an important role not only in the physiology of human and animals, but also in their metabolism.

CREATION OF EXPERIMENTAL MODEL COLITIS IN ANIMALS

New opportunities for studying inflammatory bowel disease and the effectiveness of its treatment are an urgent problem in modern biology and medicine. Animal models of IBD, in particular UC, has been used for over fifty years [88-92]. Subsequent refinement and the development of this model led to a variety of chemically-induced models [12]. These models have recently been reviewed in the context of the role of intestinal bacteria in the development of IBD [12, 91, 92].

Animal models of colitis, which can cause disease experimentally in the presence of sulfate containing compounds, are increasingly used by scientists. Additions of carrageenan, sodium lignosulfonate, and amylopectin sulfate in drinking water of guinea pigs and rabbits caused damage to the intestine which had symptoms similar to human UC [28]. The inflammation was localized distal to the cecum. In humans, the disease always occurs in the distal colon. The severity of the disease was correlated with sulfate content in the polymer. The mechanisms of these diseases are not fully understood. However, the activation of the immune response occurred in these animals after the introduction of sulfates in food. Damage to the intestinal mucosa was also observed [28, 80, 81]. The presence of carrageenan in the intestine of mice, as well as its interaction with the normal microbiota, can also cause colitis. Chronic colitis in mice and hamsters using dextran sulfate was experimental induced [5, 88].

Studies of animal models of intestinal inflammation, including ulcerative colitis in humans, show that intestinal bacteria play an important role in the initiation and maintenance of the inflammation [88, 93]. The presence of sulfate is also important in the development of these diseases [5, 71, 82]. The disruption of the qualitative and quantitative composition of the microbiota of the digestive tract may be due to infections, stress, antibiotics, chemotherapy, radiation action, poisoning, poor nutrition, and others factors [5, 71]. The changes in the composition of the intestinal microbiota in turn can cause disorders of metabolic processes and immune status, which indicates the close relationship between the host and his normal microbiome [93].

In literature, there is a lot of data on the characteristics of animal models of intestinal inflammation which was chemically created [88–92]. However, the creation of the inflammatory bowel disease using SRB has not been reported yet. To understand the more detailed contribution of sulfate and the etiological role of SRB in the development of colitis, the steps for the creation of inflammation (colitis) in animals by involving both sulfate and SRB cultures will be described below.

In this experiment, about 45 animals should be separated equally into three groups (Figure 7). The laboratory, male or female rats (about 7–8 months age and the same weight, 250 ± 25 g) were kept in standard vivarium conditions. The laboratory animals belonged to the fourth class of cleanliness by microbiological status. Their diet contained a standard certified feed for laboratory rats. All manipulations with the animals were carried out under the principles of the "European Convention for the Protection of Vertebrate Animals Used for Experimental and Other Scientific Purposes" (Strasbourg, 1986).

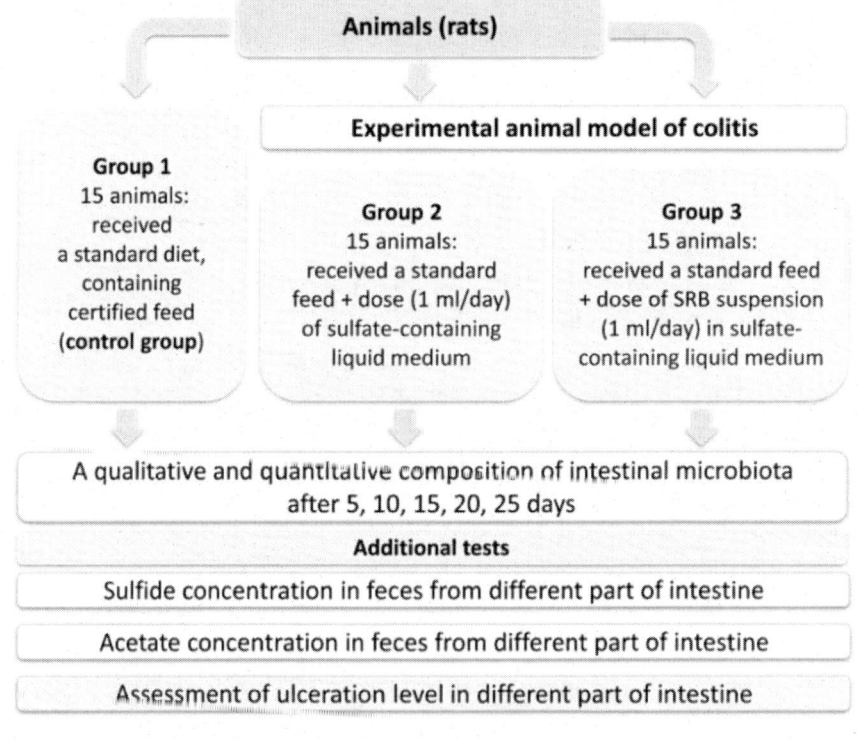

Figure 7. The scheme of the creation of inflammation (colitis) in animals.

The first group of rats received the standard diet containing the certified feed and was used as a control. The second and third groups were taken for the creation of an experimental animal model of ulcerative colitis [94]. Animals from the second group received the standard feed and a dose

(1 ml per each day) of sulfate-containing liquid medium (Postgate, without Mohr's salt) [49, 95] for the initiation of SRB's own potential microbiome. The third group of animals received the standard feed and a dose of SRB suspension in medium (1 ml per each day; the concentration of bacterial cells was 3 mg/ml). The SRB, *D. piger* Vib-7 and *D. orale* Rod-9, were previously isolated from the human large intestine and identified by sequence analysis of the 16S rRNA gene [68, 69]. GenBank access number for *D. piger* Vib-7 is KT881309.1 and *D. orale* Rod-9 is MF939896.1. The liquid Postgate medium or a suspension with SRB was orally introduced into the stomach during 25 days. The qualitative and quantitative composition of intestinal microbiome was studied in the animals of the control and experimental groups after 5, 10, 15, 20, 25 days from the beginning of injection of the medium or a SRB cell suspension. The animals were decapitated under ether anesthesia and the isolated colonic segments were selected for these studies.

Bacteriological Studies

To study the lumen microbiota of the rat colon, squeezed contents of 3-cm sized segments of the distal colon were taken by sterile forceps under sterile conditions and weighed. The weighed samples were added in a sterile tube with a tenfold volume of sterile isotonic sodium chloride solution (dilution 10^{-1}). The mixture was thoroughly triturated with a sterile glass rod to form a homogeneous mass. Subsequently, a series of tenfold dilutions (from $10^{-2}...10^{-5}$) in sterile isotonic sodium chloride solution was prepared from the homogenate. After tenfold serial dilutions in sterile isotonic sodium chloride solution, the dimensional volumes (0.1 ml) were passaged on the selective microbial culture media for each genus of *Enterobacteriacea* family. Identification of the isolated cultures of anaerobic and aerobic microorganisms was carried out by morphological, tinctirial, cultural, biochemical properties [65] using test system API 20E for identification of *Enterobacteriacea* family. The sulfate-reducing bacteria were grown in a nutrition-modified liquid medium and their identification was carried out as described previously [68]. SRB growth was evidenced by black staining (ferrous sulfide) of the medium. After cultivation, the number of colonies was counted and the population microbial level of each group of microorganisms in $\log_{10}$ colony-forming units (CFU) per gram of wet weight stool was recorded and used in calculations.

The results of these studies showed that microbiota of the first group (control) receiving the standard diet during twenty-five days, were almost unchanged. In total, fifteen genera of the bacteria were isolated in particular *Bacteroides, Prevotella, Bifidobacterium, Lactobacillus, Eubacterium, Fusobacterium, Clostridium, Peptococcus, Peptostreptococcus, Escherichia coli* (lactose-positive), *E. coli* (lactose-negative), *Proteus, Klebsiella, Enterococcus, Staphylococcus, Streptococcus, Candida*, and some SRB (Figure 8).

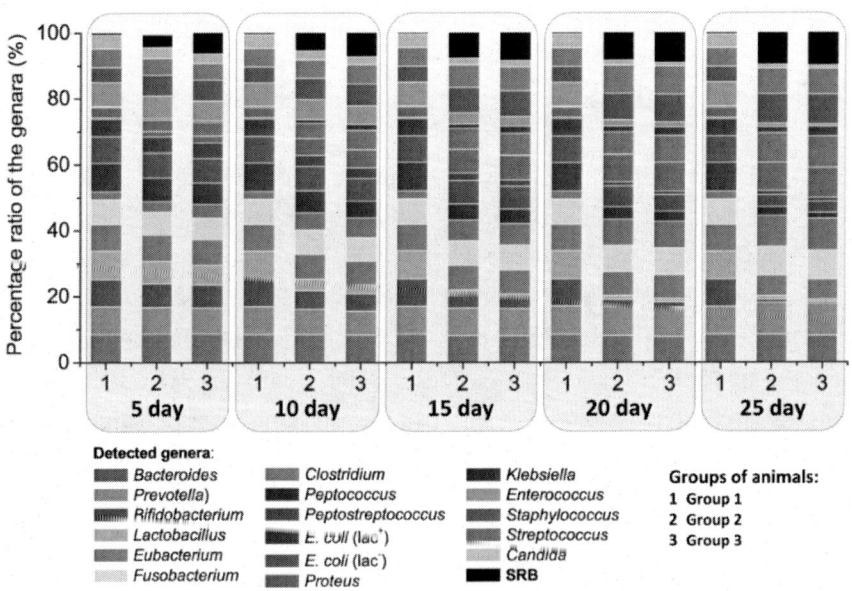

Figure 8. The microbiota of the distal colon in the rats under the effect of specific conditions during twenty-five days.

The largest number and most common of the microorganisms among these genera were detected on the fifth day ($\log_{10}$CFU/gram): *Bacteroides* (9.14 ± 0.89), *Prevotella* (9.11 ± 0.87), *Lactobacillus* (9.24 ± 0.91), *Peptococcus* (9.08 ± 0.93), and *Bifidobacterium* (8.99 ± 0.86). A slightly lower number of the intestinal bacterial genera *Eubacterium* (8.72 ± 0.85), *Fusobacterium* (8.25 ± 0.82), *Peptostreptococcus* (8.82 ± 0.78), *Enterococcus* (7.84 ± 0.74), *Streptococcus* (6.22 ± 0.63) were observed. The lowest number of the microorganisms – *E. coli* (lac$^+$) (5.61 ± 0.54), *Staphylococcus* (5.03 ± 0.47), *Candida* (4.42 ± 0.39), *Proteus* (3.24 ± 0.33), *Clostridium* (2.72 ± 0.24), *E. coli* (lac$^-$) (0.54 ± 0.051), *Klebsiella* (0.39 ± 0.035), and SRB (0.58 ± 0.055) – were isolated. The quantitative and qualitative ratio of these microorganisms was almost constant during 25 days in the first (control) group of the experimental animals [94].

Adding a dose of the modified liquid medium, which contained sulfate ions in the standard animal diet (second group) and the dose of a suspension with SRB (third group), caused changes in the microbiome that were able to be observed on the fifth day of the experiment. In this case, the injection of the medium to animals' gastrointestinal tract caused a reduction in the number of *Lactobacillus* (20%), *Peptococcus* (14%), *Candida* (21%), and an increase in number of *E. coli* (lac$^-$) (70%), *Proteus* (13%), *Klebsiella* and *Staphylococcus* (28%), and SRB (86%) in the second animal group on the fifth day. The dose of the suspension with the strains of SRB to the tract led to the reduction in the number of *Lactobacillus* (30%), *Peptococcus* (22%), *Candida* (25%), and the increase in the number of *Clostridium* (40%), *E. coli* (lac$^-$) (78%), *Proteus* (26%), *Klebsiella* (36%) and *Staphylococcus* (30%), and SRB (92%) in third animal group on the fifth day of the detection compared to the control.

As this study shows, the qualitative and quantitative changes in the intestinal microbiome depended on the time of the introduction of the dose of the sulfate containing medium or bacterial suspension. Each additional dose of the medium or the suspension caused significant alterations to the bowel microbiota in the rats on the 10th, 15th, 20th, 25th day of the detection. The greatest qualitative and quantitative changes in the microbiome in the second and third animal groups were observed on the

25th day. Under these conditions, everyday introduction of the dose of the medium or the suspension led to a significant reduction in the number of *Bifidobacterium* and *Lactobacillus* (90%), *Eubacterium* (30%), *Peptococcus* (73%), *Peptostreptococcus* (57%), *Enterococcus* (86%), *Candida* (77%), and the increase in the number of *Clostridium* (71%), *E. coli* (lac$^+$) (79%), *E. coli* (lac$^-$) (94%), *Proteus* (63%), *Klebsiella* (80%), *Staphylococcus* (43%), and SRB (95%) in the second group compared to the control on the 25th day.

A significant reduction in the number of *Lactobacillus* and *Bifidobacterium* (93–95%), *Eubacterium* (32%), *Peptococcus* (81%), *Peptostreptococcus* (62%), *Enterococcus* (91%), *Candida* (79%), and the increase in the number of *Clostridium* (73%), *E. coli* (lac$^+$) (81%), *E. coli* (lac$^-$) (96%), *Proteus* (67%), *Klebsiella* (86%), *Staphylococcus* (45%), and SRB (97%) compared to the control in the third animal group was observed on the 25th day.

One of the very important indicators of the intestinal bacteria number for characterizing the bowel conditions and its microbiota is the sustainability index (*SI*, %) and frequencies (P_i) of the microorganisms. The colon microbiota of the different animal groups on the twenty-fifth day were also assessed by Sustainability Index (*SI*, %) and detection frequencies (P_i) [94]:

$$SI = p/P \times 100, P_i = A/B$$

where **SI** is a sustainability index (%), **p** is the number of samples containing the studied bacterial strain, **P** is the total number of samples containing all isolates of the bacteria, **A** is the number of strains of the specific type and **B** is the total number of all strains.

The results of this study showed that the *SI* and P_i data were significantly different in the three groups of animals (Table 2). These data were also consistent to previously obtained results of the qualitative and quantitative changes in the microbiota in the rats on the 25th day. The predominant bacteria of the colon of the first (control) group were *Bacteroides*, *Prevotella*, *Bifidobacterium*, *Lactobacillus*, *Eubacterium*, *Fusobacterium*, *E. coli* (lac$^+$), and *Enterococcus*. These data indicated that the bacterial genera were dominant representatives of the obligate microbiota of the lumen of the distal colon in the rats. It should be also noted that the values SI and P_i for *Peptostreptococcus* genera, *Peptococcus*, and for yeast *Candida* genus were lower compared to other isolated genera. The sustainability index and the frequency of detection were also lower for *Proteus*, *Klebsiella*, *Streptococcus* and *Clostridium* genera, and SRB. Thus, these microorganisms were representatives of the facultative, transient bowel microbiota of the rats.

Table 2. Sustainability index and frequencies of the microbiota of the distal colon in the rats (data from Kushkevych 2014) [94]

Microorganisms	Groups of animals								
	Group 1			Group 2			Group 3		
	N	SI (%)	P_i	N	SI (%)	P_i	N	SI (%)	P_i
Bacteroides	25	100	0.102	30	100	0.101	28	100	0.086
Prevotella	15	60	0.062	18	65	0.061	21*	70	0.065
Bifidobacterium	24	100	0.099	7***	10***	0.024***	4***	8***	0.012***
Lactobacillus	28	100	0.115	9**	14***	0.033***	6***	11***	0.018***
Eubacterium	22	80	0.091	26	75	0.087	24	85	0.074
Fusobacterium	15	55	0.062	17	58	0.057	19	60	0.059
Clostridium	4	15	0.016	15***	60***	0.051***	18***	77***	0.056***
Peptococcus	11	40	0.045	8*	25*	0.027*	6*	21*	0.018**
Peptostreptococcus	9	45	0.037	7	23*	0.021*	2***	17**	0.006***
E. coli (lac⁺)	23	90	0.095	25	95	0.084	21	100	0.065*
E. coli (lac⁻)	3	10	0.012	21***	98***	0.071***	25***	100***	0.077***
Proteus	8	30	0.033	17**	67**	0.057**	26***	82**	0.080***
Klebsiella	2	5	0.008	8***	29***	0.027***	10***	42***	0.031***
Enterococcus	21	100	0.086	25	100	0.084	22	100	0.068
Staphylococcus	15	100	0.062	19	100	0.064	25*	100	0.079
Streptococcus	5	60	0.021	13**	93*	0.044**	27***	98**	0.083***
Candida	8	35	0.033	6	50*	0.020*	10	72*	0.031
SRB	5	33	0.021	25***	100***	0.084***	30***	100***	0.093***

Comment: N is the number of the isolated strains; SI is the sustainability index; P_i is frequencies. Data were calculated for intestinal microbiota on the 25th day. The statistical significance of the values M ± m, n = 3; * $P < 0.05$, ** $P < 0.01$, *** $P < 0.001$, compared to first (control) group.

Significant changes in the qualitative and quantitative microbial composition of the colon in the second and third animals groups were observed. The most noticeable changes were specific to genera *Bifidobacterium, Lactobacillus, Clostridium, Peptococcus, Peptostreptococcus, E. coli* (lac⁻), *Proteus, Klebsiella, Staphylococcus, Streptococcus*, and SRB for animals of the second group. Similar results of the sustainability index and frequencies of the microbiota of the third animal group were obtained for the following genera: *Bifidobacterium, Lactobacillus, Clostridium, Peptococcus, Peptostreptococcus, E. coli* (lac⁻), *Proteus, Klebsiella, Staphylococcus, Streptococcus*, and the SRB. Thus, the most significant changes were characteristic for the following genera *Bifidobacterium, Lactobacillus, Clostridium, Peptococcus, Peptostreptococcus, E. coli* (both lac⁺ and lac⁻), *Proteus, Klebsiella, Staphylococcus, Streptococcus*, and SRB [94].

Sulfide Concentration

Colonic microbiota, including SRB, can produce large quantities of hydrogen sulfide [5, 96]. *In vitro* studies indicate that fecal bacteria liberate hydrogen sulfide far more efficiently from organic sulfur-containing compounds than from sulfate [96, 97]. After 5, 10, 15, 20, 25 days from the beginning of injection of the medium or a SRB suspension, fresh fecal samples from different sections of the large intestine were passed into preweighed containers: 20-ml polypropylene syringes for measurement of H_2S release; pre-weighed 50-ml test tubes containing 5 ml of 2% zinc acetate (ice cold) for H_2S and acetate concentration measurements; and 4-ml vials for SRB culture [97]. The following collection of the fecal sample, the plunger was immediately reinserted into the syringe, the gas space was flushed with nitrogen (N_2), 20 ml of N_2 was added, and the syringe was sealed with a stopcock. The syringes were incubated at +37°C, and at 1, 2, 4, and 24 h the gas volume was recorded and a 0.3-ml gas sample was removed for analysis for H_2S. At 24 h, the syringes were weighed and fecal weight was determined by the difference. The rate of release of H_2S per gram of wet weight was calculated from the concentration of H_2S, the volume of the gas space, and fecal weight [97, 98].

The vial containing the fecal sample and zinc acetate was weighed and fecal weight was determined by the difference. The volume of zinc acetate was adjusted to give a 1:100 ratio of feces to zinc acetate and the sample was homogenized. A 0.5-ml aliquot of the homogenate was added to a 20-ml polypropylene syringe, 0.5 ml of 12 N HCl was instilled into the syringe, and the syringe was sealed with a stopcock. After 30 min, a 0.3-ml aliquot of gas space was analyzed for H_2S [97, 98].

The SRB *Desulfovibrio* and *Desulfomicrobium* genera, oxidize organic compounds incompletely to acetate [5, 49, 65]. The oxidation of lactate to acetate occurs together with the concurrent reduction of sulfate to sulfide [5, 14]. Sulfide and acetate concentration in the fecal samples from different sections of the large intestine of the rats – in particular the caecum, ascending colon, transverse colon, descending colon, and the rectum – was determined [94]. The results of these studies showed that the level of sulfide in the feces of the first group (control) during the 25 days was almost unchanged (Table 3).

The concentration of sulfide and acetate in fecal samples from different sections of the large intestine was slightly different from each other. The values of concentration (μmole per gram and mmole per gram, respectively) in the fecal samples from the caecum (2.08 ± 0.19 and 16.10 ± 1.53), ascending colon (2.31 ± 0.21 and 17.88 ± 1.74), transverse colon (2.45 ± 0.23 and 18.96 ± 1.81), descending colon (2.49 ± 0.22 and 19.27±1.88), and the rectum (2.43 ± 0.24 and 18.81 ± 1.79) were determined on the fifth day for sulfide and acetate, respectively. The quantitative ratio of these compounds was almost constant during twenty-five days in the first group of the experimental animals [94].

Significant changes in the concentration of sulfide and acetate in all sections of the large intestine in the second and third groups of rats on the fifth day of the experiment were already observed. The highest level of sulfide and acetate was accumulated in the descending colon of the second and third groups during the 25 days [94]. In this case, sulfide and acetate concentration increased directly proportionally to the duration of introduction of the dose of the medium or the suspension with SRB. The values of sulfide and acetate concentration in the fecal samples from descending colon increased respectively in the second and third groups of rats by 32 and 65% as well as 35 and 69% compared to the control on the 5th day. More significant quantitative changes in the concentration of these compounds and their substantial increase were observed on the 25th day. Under these conditions, the level of sulfide and acetate in the descending colon increased respectively by 88 and 95% in the second group as well as 93 and 97% in the third group of animals [94].

The correlation and systematic statistical analysis between the parameters of sulfide and acetate accumulation in the descending colon in the animal groups during 25 days was carried out. A strong inversely positive correlation between sulfide and acetate accumulation was demonstrated in the paper [94]. The results of the systematic statistical analysis showed that the variance, pooled variance, t-statistics in the experimental groups of animals were quite variable on the 25th day of the detection. These statistical parameters also depended on the duration of the experiment. However, t critical one-way (1.860 ± 0.181) and t critical two-way (2.306 ± 0.224) were similar for each of the parameters.

Sulfide exists in ionized, non-volatile states (S^- or HS^-), as well as volatile H_2S [28]. Levitt et al. (1999) have shown that about 95% of the sulfide produced in the gut is absorbed and the vast majority of the 5% passed in feces is tightly bound to other compounds [99]. Hence, fecal sulfide concentration appears to reflect sulfide binding capacity rather than intraluminal production [97]. Hydrogen sulfide's volatile thiol binds to the heme moiety of cytochrome a_3, blocking the terminal step in electron transport [100]. When administered systemically, H_2S has a median lethal dose (LD_{50}) for rodents similar to that of cyanide [97]. The volatility of H_2S results in its rapid dissociation from fecal material; and this gas has very high tissue permeability [101]. Thus, the colonocytes are exposed to virtually the entire bacterial output of this compound, in contrast to other potentially toxic bacterial metabolites, which remain in the feces or which have low permeability for the colonic mucosa [97]. While the colonocytes efficiently detoxifies H_2S via conversion to thiosulfate [98, 99], there has been speculation that this highly toxic compound could play a pathogenic role in colonic diseases, particularly UC [102].

Table 3. Sulfide concentration in fecal samples from different sections of the large intestine of the rats (data from Kushkevych 2014) [94]

Groups of animals	Section of the intestine	Time of detection (days)				
		5th	10th	15th	20th	25th
		H$_2$S concentration (µmole per gram)				
Group 1	Caecum	2.06	2.08	1.78	2.03	1.88
	Ascending colon	2.29	2.31	2.01	2.26	2.11
	Transverse colon	2.43	2.45	2.15	2.40	2.25
	Descending colon	2.47	2.49	2.19	2.44	2.29
	Rectum	2.41	2.43	2.13	2.38	2.23
Average		2.33 ± 0.16	2.35 ± 0.16	2.05 ± 0.16	2.30 ± 0.16	2.15 ± 0.16
Group 2	Caecum	2.23	11.15	15.61	20.07	22.76
	Ascending colon	2.72	13.60	19.04	24.48	26.64
	Transverse colon	3.23	16.15	22.61	29.07	33.76
	Descending colon	3.65	18.25	25.55	32.85	35.80
	Rectum	3.43	17.15	24.01	30.87	32.16
Average		3.05 ± 0.57	15.26 ± 2.87	21.36 ± 4.02	27.47 ± 5.17	30.22 ± 5.38
Group 3	Caecum	4.27	27.87	29.89	30.43	31.24
	Ascending colon	5.43	34.03	37.98	40.83	42.10
	Transverse colon	6.39	40.38	44.71	49.49	52.65
	Descending colon	7.60	45.63	53.17	60.36	61.14
	Rectum	7.16	42.88	50.10	56.42	56.42
Average		6.17 ± 1.34	38.16 ± 7.18	43.17 ± 9.40	47.51 ± 12.09	48.71 ± 12.02

Sulfide also has been linked to colon neoplasia via the observation that sulfide exposure induced proliferation in the upper crypt region of the colonic mucosa [103-105], a finding associated with mucosal hyperplasia [97]. Hydrogen sulfide is a highly toxic compound that has a median lethal concentration on the same order of magnitude as that of cyanide [106]. The potential for local toxicity of sulfide in the colon has been studied by Roediger et al. [103,104], who incubated human and rat colonic epithelial cells with a range of sulfide concentrations [105]. Low concentrations of sulfide inhibited butyrate oxidation, whereas higher concentrations caused inhibition of glucose oxidation. Of interest are studies showing that colonic mucosal biopsy specimens from people with moderately severe UC similarly demonstrate inhibition of butyrate oxidation with preservation of glucose metabolism [102, 105]. In people with severe colitis, both reactions are altered. In animals, inhibition of fatty acid oxidation via rectal instillation of sodium 2-bromo-octanoate produced a colitis resembling UC [28].

Hydrogen sulfide produced by colonic SRB can be toxic and involved in the pathogenesis of IBD, including UC. Colonic sulfide exposure has previously been assessed via measurements of fecal sulfide concentration [99]. Levitt et al. has shown that 1% of fecal sulfide in rats was free, the remainder being bound in soluble and insoluble complexes. Thus fecal sulfide concentrations may reflect sulfide binding capacity rather than the toxic potential of feces [98, 99].

The colonic bacteria ferment unabsorbed carbohydrates, producing the acetic, propionic and n-butyric acids [107]. Vogt et al. has shown that the mean percentage of butyrate absorption (30.2 ± 4.6%) exceeded that of acetate (24.1 ± 3.7%). The fecal molar acetate percentage was inversely correlated with the percentage of acetate absorption. There was no combination effect on short chain fatty acids absorption, and the chain-length effect suggests passive diffusion as a likely mechanism of absorption. Furthermore, fecal acetate may reflect absorption, rather than the production of colonic acetate [107].

The level of ulcerations of different sections of the large intestine in rats of the first and second experimental groups under the effect of specific conditions during 25 days was evaluated (Table 4). Ulceration on the fifth day was not detected. However, ulcers began to form by the 10th day. The highest level of ulceration on the 25th day in both animal groups was observed. In this case, the largest number of ulcers was found in the descending colon compared to other parts of the large intestine in the rats. The data on level of ulcerations in the descending colon are consistent with the results that hydrogen sulfide and acetate accumulation. It was also highest in the descending colon. Comparing the ulcer formation level in both animal groups, the higher level of ulcerations was observed in the third group than the second animal group. Perhaps, the SRB *D. piger* Vib-7 and *D. orale* Rod-9 are more aggressive for the large intestine and can be involved in much more intense IBD development, including colitis [94].

Table 4. The level of ulcerations in the second and third groups of animals under the specific conditions (data from Kushkevych 2014) [94]

Groups of animals	Section of the intestine	Time of detection (days)				
		5th	10th	15th	20th	25th
Group 2	Caecum	ND	ND	5 ± 0.49	9 ± 0.88	18 ± 1.76
	Ascending colon	ND	ND	12 ± 1.18	14 ± 1.37	24 ± 2.35
	Transverse colon	ND	5 ± 0.47	14 ± 1.33	17 ± 1.62	27 ± 2.84
	Descending colon	ND	7 ± 0.69	17 ± 1.67	20 ± 1.96	29 ± 3.24
	Rectum	ND	6 ± 0.59	15 ± 1.47	22 ± 2.16	26 ± 2.75
Group 3	Caecum	ND	nd	11 ± 1.06**	22 ± 2.12**	51 ± 4.90***
	Ascending colon	ND	8 ± 0.77	27 ± 2.62**	33 ± 3.17**	68 ± 6.54***
	Transverse colon	ND	13 ± 1.25**	32 ± 3.08**	48 ± 4.62***	71 ± 6.83**
	Descending colon	ND	18 ± 1.73**	39 ± 3.75**	53 ± 5.10***	78 ± 7.50***
	Rectum	ND	15 ± 1.44**	34 ± 3.27**	52 ± 4.94**	76 ± 7.21***

Comment: The level of ulcerations was assessed visually and expressed as a percentage of the number and size of ulcers per cm^2 of the intestine; "ND" is not detected. The statistical significance of the values: M ± m, n = 3; ** $P < 0.01$, *** $P < 0.001$, compared to the second animals group.

Studies comparing the number of SRB and their products in feces from patients with colitis as well as normal subjects have yielded varying results. One report found that people with ulcerative colitis had a 70%

higher stool sulfide concentration, a twofold increase in the sulfide production rate and a fivefold increase in the SRB [12].

One research group found no increase in total fecal SRB; however, UC feces contained different ratios of the various species of SRB. The bacteria of UC subjects were more active and grew better in a confined area [34, 35]. In addition, those with colitis had a 28% increase in fecal sulfide levels and more than a doubling in sulfide production rates. Another study found no difference in the fecal SRB of UC subjects versus that of healthy controls [96]. It should be also noted that the microbiota of the lumen of the distal colon (microbial number, their ratio, the sustainability index and frequency of detection) was significantly changed in the second and third groups. These groups had received the dose with sulfate containing medium or the *D. piger* Vib-7 and *D. orale* Rod-9 compared to the control group [94]. Under these conditions, the number of *Bifidobacterium* and *Lactobacillus* genera significantly decreased, while the number of *Clostridium*, *Escherichia*, *Proteus*, *Klebsiella*, *Staphylococcus* genera, and the SRB were significantly increased. Perhaps, these microorganisms play a major role in the development of IBD, including UC.

The presence of *E coli* in patients with ulcerative colitis was investigated, and it was reported that *E coli* could be detected only in a small proportion of tissue samples [108, 109]. Studies on mucosal adhesion of pathogenic bacteria in ulcerative colitis are controversial. A significantly enhanced adhesion of isolates of *E. coli* from stool specimens and rectal biopsies from ulcerative colitis patients to buccal epithelial cells was found in comparison with patients with infectious diarrhea or normal controls [110]. The adhesive properties were similar to those of pathogenic intestinal *E coli*, suggesting that virulent *E coli* strains might participate in the pathogenesis of UC [111, 112]. Another study reported adherence of only *E. coli* subtypes to rectal mucosa, however, no differences in adhesion could be found between UC patients and controls [113, 114]. Using a hybridization *in situ* technique, a significantly higher number of bacteria were found within the mucus layer and not adherent to the surface of the epithelium in ulcerative colitis patients compared with controls, independently from the degree of inflammation. Most likely the bacteria belong to a variety of species, considering the broad specificity of the probe used in this study [115]. To summarize, there is incomplete information and continuing controversy about the role, adherent properties, and subtypes of *E coli* which might be important in the pathogenesis of ulcerative colitis [110].

M. Campieri and P. Gionchetti (2001) have reported that the role of bacteria in pathogenesis was shown most convincingly in animal models [110]. A causative role for *Bacteroides* species in experimental ulcerative colitis was suggested. In a carrageenan guinea pig model of experimental colitis, germ free animals did not develop colitis until after monoassociation with *Bacteroides vulgatus* [116]. Subsequently, it was suggested that different strains of *B. vulgatus* led to considerable differences in the inflammatory response without correlation between the sources of strains and the severity of carrageenan induced lesions. In this model, pretreatment with metronidazole prevented colitis, while administration of Gram positive organisms or coliforms was not effective. These data suggest the need for an interaction between bacteria sensitive to metronidazole and dietary sulfate. More recently, the degree of caecal inflammation in HLA-B27 transgenic rats was shown to be correlated with levels of isolates on *Bacteroides* selective medium and increased anaerobic/aerobic and *Bacteroides*/aerobic ratios [117]. Indirect evidence for the interaction between luminal flora and the immune system exists from studies using animal models with disruptions in immunoregulatory molecules. It was reported that spontaneous colitis, which consistently develops in knockout and transgenic mucin models, does not occur when these mice are maintained in germ free conditions [118, 119].

Fite et al. (2013) has shown that the bacteria belonging to the normal colonic microbiota were associated with the etiology of UC. Although several mucosal species have been implicated in the disease process, the organisms and the mechanisms involved are unknown [120]. These authors have also characterized mucosal biofilm communities over time and determined the relationship of these bacteria to patient age, disease severity, and duration. Multiple rectal biopsy specimens were taken from 33 patients with active ulcerative colitis over a period of one year.

Real-time PCR was used to quantify mucosal bacteria in ulcerative colitis patients compared to 18 non IBD controls, and the relationship between indicators of disease severity and bacterial colonization was evaluated by linear regression analysis. Significant differences in bacterial populations were detected among the UC mucosa and control group, which varied over the study period. High clinical activity indices and sigmoidoscopy scores were associated with enterobacteria, desulfovibrios, type E *Clostridium perfringens* and *Enterococcus faecalis*, whereas the reverse was true for *Clostridium butyricum*, *Ruminococcus albus*, and *Eubacterium rectale*. Bacteria *Lactobacillus* and *Bifidobacterium* numbers were linked with low clinical activity indices. Only *E. rectale* and *Clostridium clostridioforme* had high age dependence. These findings demonstrated that longitudinal variations in mucosal bacterial populations occur in UC and that bacterial community structure was related to disease severity [120].

In recent years, there have been many reports about using animal models to investigate drugs for IBD. Acetic acid-induced damage of colonic mucosa is often used as the experimental animal model. Zheng et al. (2000) have investigated the use of this animal model by administering various concentrations of trinitrobenzenesulfonic acid [90].

The specific pathogenesis underlying IBD is complex, and it is even more difficult to decipher the pathophysiology to explain for the similarities and differences between two of its major subtypes, Crohn's disease and UC. Low et al. (2013) has reported the therapeutic strategies and approaches tested on UC animal models. UC is an idiopathic chronic relapsing-remitting inflammatory disorder that affects the colon, characterized by diarrhea and rectal bleeding [89]. The molecular etiology of ulcerative colitis development is complex and involves genetic, microbial, environmental, and other unknown factors. The discussion of the underlying pathophysiology of UC and how observations from animal models that mimic UC contribute to a better understanding of this disease as well as lead to advancement in novel treatment design was also reported by Low et al. (2013). There has been a steady increase in the global incidence of UC. Currently, the prevalence in Europe and North America is 24.3 and 19.2 per 100,000 individuals, respectively, and 6.3 per 100,000 people in Asia and the Middle East. Most patients develop UC between the ages of 15 and 30 years, although individuals aged 50–70 years form another potential risk group. There are no significant differences in ulcerative colitis risk between sexes. The growing prevalence of this disease increases both economic and health care burdens [89]. Animal models of IBD have significant advantages – one can investigate not only the factors concerned in pathogenesis, but also the secondary effects of ulceration, e.g., liver changes, effects on protein metabolism, electrolytic changes in the cellular and extracellular spaces, and other systemic complications [29, 92].

Barnet et al. (2011) have reported that these animal models may also be used to study the influence of drugs or other potential therapies in the pathogenesis and course of the disease process. However, none of the current IBD models in itself constitutes a faithful equivalent for the human diseases. It may therefore be essential to evaluate the effect of any candidate therapies in several IBD models. The wide variety of models of IBD includes chemically-induced models, adoptive transfer models, and genetically modified models such as gene knockouts and transgenic animals [92]. There is clearly still a role for animal models of the IBD. However more appropriate use of new information and technologies, better classification of IBD based on both phenotypic and genetic information, and closer alliances between fundamental biological researchers and clinicians are required to ensure that the key lessons from these models are effectively moved into clinical practice. This should enable more successful strategies for the prevention and amelioration of this debilitating condition [92].

Based on all obtained results in these studies, it can be concluded that injection of the sulfate containing medium or suspension with SRB in the gastrointestinal tract of the rats caused significant changes in the microbiota of the animals during the 25 day experiment. Under these conditions, the structure of the microbiota, the number of microorganisms, their ratio, sustainability index, and frequency on the 25th day were significantly changed in both experimental groups of the animals. The number of *Bifidobacterium, Lactobacillus, Peptostreptococcus,* and *Peptococcus* genera was decreased. The number of *Clostridium*, *Escherichia*, *Staphylococcus*, *Proteus* genera, and SRB were increased. There was significant colonization by the *Escherichia* (lac⁻) and *Klebsiella* genera in the lumen of the colon. The highest level of sulfide and acetate accumulation in the feces was detected on the 25th day. Sulfide and acetate concentration increased directly proportionally to the duration of injection of the dose of the sulfate containing medium or the suspension with the SRB. However, significantly increased concentration of these compounds was observed in the fecal samples from the third group compared to the second group of the animals, which reserved only the sulfate containing medium. These data were consistent with the results of the ulcerations in the third group where the level of ulcer formation was much higher than the second group. The contribution of SRB injected in the gastrointestinal tract was significantly more than endogenous intestinal microbiota.

Thus, the injection of the sulfate containing medium or suspension with the SRB in the gastrointestinal tract of the rats leads to a change in the qualitative and quantitative composition of the intestinal microbiota (dysbiosis) which may be a result of the development of the IBD, including UC, and various pathological processes. These studies might help in predicting the development of the diseases of the gastrointestinal tract, by providing further details on the etiology of bowel diseases which are very important for the clinical diagnosis of these disease types. Understanding the role of intestinal SRB in colonic conditions could be enhanced by the ability to inhibit the number of the SRB and/or reduce the production of hydrogen sulfide and acetate. This would help to clarify the factors influencing sulfide production in the human colon.

GENERALIZATION OF THE RESEARCHES

Sulfate content in food and beverages varies greatly and depends on their type. Foods rich in sulfate can be both vegetarian and animal origin. The Western diet contains 1.6 mmol of sulfate per day and the African diet 2.7 mmol of sulfate per day. Moreover, another source of sulfate in the intestine can be food additives, which preserve flavor or enhance its taste, appearance, or other qualities.

Absorption of sulfate in the intestine can be genetically determined and can differ in people. There is a maximum sulfate absorption of 16 mmol per day in normal individuals. Up to 9 mmol per day of sulfate reached colon and less than 0.5 mmol per day was excreted in the feces [13]. Probably, such a low concentration of sulfate in the bowel lumen may be sufficient for the growth of SRB. The diet and intestinal absorption are obviously the key factors determining the concentration of sulfate in the lumen colon.

Free sulfate ions presented in the intestinal lumen are reduced in two ways; the first, in the process of assimilation sulfate reduction, and in the second case by the SRB in the process of dissimilatory sulfate reduction. In the assimilatory sulfate reduction, sulfate is used for for biosynthetic processes as a source of sulfur (e.g., the synthesis of sulfur-containing amino acids or other organic compounds). The second is by the dissimilatory sulfate reduction process which is carried out by intestinal SRB. In this case, sulfate is used as a terminal electron acceptor and reduced to toxic hydrogen sulfide. The SRB can use sulfite, thiosulfate or other oxidized sulfur compounds, except sulfate, as an electron acceptor and reduce them to hydrogen sulfide in the dissimilatory sulfate reduction process. The intestinal species of *Desulfovibrio* genus are the most often isolated among all SRB both from healthy subjects and from patients with various diseases.

The addition of sulfate-containing medium and a suspension of SRB to the digestive tract of rats caused the occurrence of colitis. These data confirmed the important role of sulfate and the contribution of SRB to the development of inflammatory bowel disease (Figure 9).

On the other hand, the increased number of SRB can affect the process of methanogenesis, suppressing methanogenic microorganisms by the production of hydrogen sulfide. Obviously, the amount of SRB in intestinal lumen can depend not only on the presence of sulfate in food, but can be also associated with human populations.

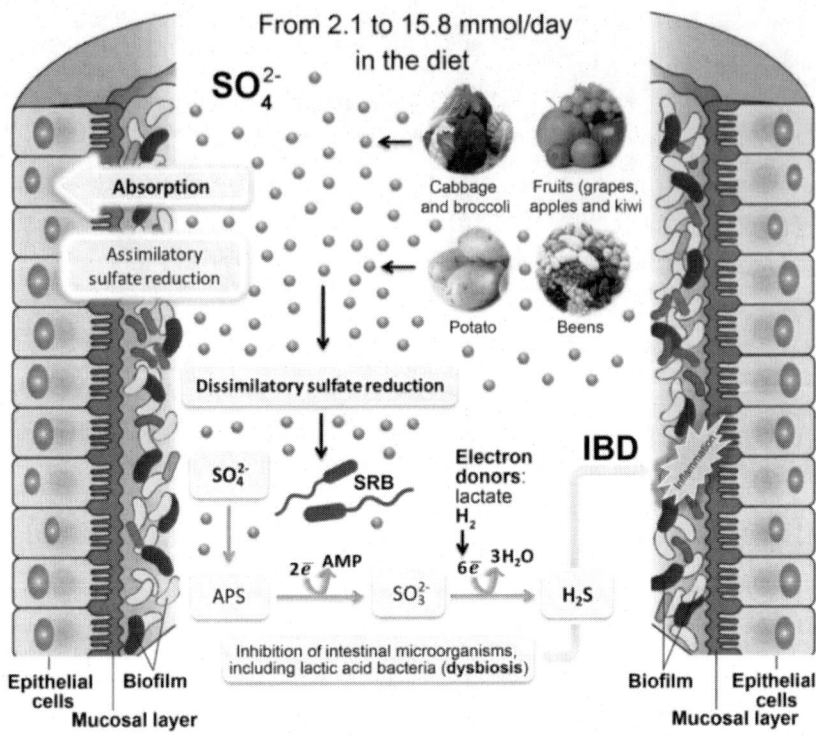

Figure 9. Generalization scheme of sulfate role in the colitis development.

The main factors affecting the development of colitis:

- diet and the content of sulfate in food and beverages;
- absorption capacity of the intestine (genetically determined, different for every individual);
- presence of free sulfate in the intestine;
- SRB increased quantity, respectively, increased production of hydrogen sulfide;
- the effect of hydrogen sulfide on the intestinal microbiota, inhibition of lactic acid bacteria, and other microorganisms (dysbiosis).
- because of dysbiosis, other intestinal microorganisms can be involved in the process of ulceration and colitis development.

It should be also noted that SRB are presented in mucosal biofilms. The physiological and biochemical properties of SRB in the intestinal lumen and in the composition of the biofilm may differ. Intestinal SRB have an effect on the human physiological functions and health. That's why, the investigation of the SRB, the process of dissimilatory sulfate reduction, production of hydrogen sulfide, and their role in the IBD in animals and humans should increasingly attract the attention of scientists. It is also important to investigate the activity of the newly synthesized compounds [121-123] against on the growth of SRB and their process of sulfate reduction.

The described physiological and biochemical parameters are important for a more detailed understanding of sulfate dissimilation in the human and animal's bowel, as well as studying the mechanisms of action of the antimicrobial prophylactics and the therapy against specific components involved in the pathogenesis of the disease. It is also essential for understanding the mechanisms of bowel diseases and for evaluating the effectiveness of its therapy.

ACKNOWLEDGMENTS

The author expresses gratitude to Dr. Dani Dordević, M.Sc., Ph.D. from the Department of Plant Origin Foodstuffs Hygiene and Technology, Faculty of Veterinary Hygiene and Ecology, University of Veterinary and Pharmaceutical Sciences Brno (Czech Republic) for his advice on food products and assistance during writing one of these subchapters. Also, author would like to say thank you to Lauren Cooper from California State University, Monterey Bay (USA) for her reading and grammatical corrections to this chapter.

This study was supported by Grant Agency of the Masaryk University (MUNI/A/0902/2018).

REFERENCES

[1] Burisch, J., Jess, T., Martinato, M., Lakatos, P. L. & ECCO EpiCom. (2013). The burden of inflammatory bowel disease in Europe. *J Crohns Colitis*, 7, 322–337.

[2] Frolkis, A., Dieleman, L. A., Barkema, H., et al. (2013). Environment and the inflammatory bowel diseases. *Can J Gastroenterol*, 27, 18–24.

[3] Ng, S. C., Shi, H. Y., Hamidi, N., Underwood, F. E., Tang, W., Benchimol, E. I., Panaccione, R., Ghosh, S., Wu, J. C., Chan, F. K. & Sung, J. J. (2017). Worldwide incidence and prevalence of inflammatory bowel disease in the 21st century: a systematic review of population-based studies. *The Lancet*, 390, 2769–2778.

[4] da Silva, B. C., Lyra, A. C., Rocha, R. & Santana, G. O. (2014). Epidemiology, demographic characteristics and prognostic predictors of ulcerative colitis. *World Journal of Gastroenterology*, 20(28), 9458.

[5] Kushkevych, I. V. (2016). Dissimilatory sulfate reduction in the intestinal sulfate-reducing bacteria. *Studia Biologica*, 10(1), 197–228.

[6] Kováč, J., Vítězová, M., Kushkevych, I. (2018). Metabolic activity of sulfate-reducing bacteria from rodents with colitis. *Open Med*, 13, 344–349.

[7] Kushkevych, I., Vítězová, M., Fedrová, P., et al. (2017). Kinetic properties of growth of intestinal sulphate-reducing bacteria isolated from healthy mice and mice with ulcerative colitis. *Acta Vet Brno*, 86, 405–411.

[8] Kushkevych, I., Fafula, R., Parak, T., et al. (2015). Activity of Na^+/K^+-activated Mg^{2+}-dependent ATP hydrolase in the cell-free extracts of the sulfate-reducing bacteria *Desulfovibrio piger* Vib-7 and *Desulfomicrobium* sp. Rod-9. *Acta Vet Brno*, 84, 3–12.

[9] Kushkevych, I. V. (2015). Activity and kinetic properties of phosphotrans-acetylase from intestinal sulfate-reducing bacteria. *Acta Biochemica Polonica*, 62, 1037–108.

[10] Kushkevych, I. V. (2015). Kinetic Properties of Pyruvate Ferredoxin Oxidoreductase of Intestinal Sulfate-Reducing Bacteria *Desulfovibrio piger* Vib-7 and *Desulfomicrobium* sp. Rod-9. *Polish J Microbiol*, *64*, 107–114.
[11] Florin, T. H., Neale, G., Goretski, S., et al. (1993). Sulfate in food and beverages. *J Food Compos and Anal*, *6*, 140–151.
[12] Florin, T. H. J., Gibson, G. R., Neale, G., et al. (1990). A role for sulfate-reducing bacteria in ulcerative colitis?" *Gastroenterology*, *98*, A170.
[13] Florin, T., Neale, G., Gibson, G. R., Christl, S. U. & Cummings, J. H. (1991). Metabolism of dietary sulphate: absorption and excretion in humans. *Gut*, *32*(7), 766–773.
[14] Barton, L. L. & Hamilton, W. A. (2010). *Sulphate-Reducing Bacteria. Environm. and Engin. Syst.*, Cambridge University Press, Cambridge, 553 p.
[15] Kushkevych, I., Dordević, D. & Vítězová, M. (2019). Toxicity of hydrogen sulfide toward sulfate-reducing bacteria *Desulfovibrio piger* Vib-7. *Archives of Microbiology*, *201*(3), 389–397.
[16] Kushkevych, I., Dordević, D., Vítězová, M. & Kollár, P. (2018) Cross-correlation analysis of the *Desulfovibrio* growth parameters of intestinal species isolated from people with colitis. *Biologia*, *73*, 1137–1143.
[17] Kushkevych, I., Dordević, D. & Vítězová, M. (2019). Analysis of pH dose-dependent growth of sulfate-reducing bacteria. *Open Medicine*, *14*(1), 66–74.
[18] Kushkevych, I., Dordević, D. & Kollar, P. (2018). Analysis of physiological parameters of *Desulfovibrio* strains from individuals with colitis. *Open Life Sciences*, *13*, 481–488.
[19] NAS. (1972). *Food ingredients*. Washington, DC, National Academy of Sciences, Subcommittee on Research of GRAS (Generally Recognised As Safe) List (Phase II) (DHEW No. FDA 70–22).
[20] Commission Regulation (EU) No 59/2014 of 23 January 2014.
[21] EFSA Panel on Food additives and Nutrient Sources added to Food (ANS). (2016). Scientific Opinion on the re-evaluation of sulfur

dioxide (E 220), sodium sulfite (E221), sodium bisulfite (E222), sodium metabisulfite (E223), potassium metabisulfite (E224), calcium sulfite (E226), calcium bisulfite (E227) and potassium bisulfite (E228) as food additives. *EFSA Journal*, *14*(4), 4438.
[22] Anonymous. Bread &flour regulations. London: HMSO, 1984.
[23] Freeman, G. G. & Mossadeghi, N. (1972). Studies on sulphur nutrition, flavour and allyl isothiocyanate formation in *Brassica juncea* (L.) coss. and czern.(brown mustard). *Journal of the Science of Food and Agriculture*, *23*(11), 1335–1345.
[24] Josefsson, E. (1970). Glucosinolate content and amino acid composition of rapeseed (*Brassica napus*) meal as affected by sulphur and nitrogen nutrition. *Journal of the Science of Food and Agriculture*, *21*(2), 98–103.
[25] Zoeteman, B. C. J. (1980). *Sensory assessment of water quality*. New York, NY, Pergamon Press.
[26] Greenwood, N. N. & Earnshaw, A. (1984). *Chemistry of the elements*. Oxford, Pergamon Press.
[27] McGuire, M. J., Jones, R. M., Means, E. G., Izaguirre, G. & Preston, A. E. (1984). Controlling Attached Blue-Green Algae With Copper Sulfate. *Journal-American Water Works Association*, *76*(5), 60–65.
[28] Pitcher, M. C. & Cummings, J. H. (1996). Hydrogen sulphide: a bacterial toxin in ulcerative colitis? *Gut*, *39*, 1–4.
[29] Rowan, F. E., Docherty, N. G., Coffey, J. C. & O'Connell, P. R. (2009). Sulphate-reducing bacteria and hydrogen sulphide in the aetiology of ulcerative colitis. *British Journal of Surgery: Incorporating European Journal of Surgery and Swiss Surgery*, *96*(2), 151–158.
[30] Franklin, C. A., Burnett, R. T., Paolini, R. J. & Raizenne, M. E. (1985). Health risks from acid rain: a Canadian perspective. *Environmental health perspectives*, *63*, 155–168.
[31] Cummings, J. H., Macfarlane, G. T. & Macfarlane, S. (2003). Intestinal Bacteria and Ulcerative Colitis. *Curr Issues Intest Microbiol*, *4*, 9–20.

[32] Chochetto, D. M. & Levy, G. (1981). Absorption of orally administered sodium sulphate in humans. *Pharm Sci*, *70*, 331–333.
[33] Wesley, A., Forstner, J., Qureshi, R., Mantle, M. & Forstner, G. (1983). Human intestinal mucin in cystic fibrosis. *Pediatric research*, *17*(1), 65–69.
[34] Gibson, G. R., Cummings, J. H. & Macfarlane, G. T. (1991). Growth and activities of sulphate-reducing bacteria in gut contents of health subjects and patients with ulcerative colitis. *FEMS Microbiol Ecol*, *86*, 103–112.
[35] Gibson, G. R., Macfarlane, G. T. & Cummings, J. H. (1993). Sulphate-reducing bacteria and hydrogen metabolism in the human large intestine. *Gut*, *34*, 437–439.
[36] Madigan, M. T., Martinko, J. M. & Brock, T. D. (2006). *Brock biology of microorganisms.* Upper Saddle River, NJ: Pearson Prentice Hall, 1032 p.
[37] Kushkevych, I. V., Antonyak, H. L. & Bartoš, M. (2014). Kinetic properties of adenosine triphosphate sulfurylase of intestinal sulfate-reducing bacteria. *The Ukrainian biochemical journal*, *86*(6), 129–138.
[38] Kushkevych, I. V. (2014). Kinetic characteristics of pyrophosphatase of the sulfate-reducing bacteria from human intestine. *Visnyk Lviv Uni. Biol. Series*, *68*, 158–166.
[39] Sperling, D., Kappler, U., Wynen, A., Dahl, C. & Truper, H. (1998). Dissimilatory ATP sulfurylase from the hyperthermophilic sulphate reducer *Archaeoglobus fulgidus* belongs to the group of homo-oligomeric ATP sulfurylases. *FEMS Microbiol Lett*, *162*, 257–264.
[40] Ravilious, G. E., Herrmann, J., Lee, S. G., Westfall, C. S., Jez, J. M. (2013). Kinetic mechanism of the dimeric ATP sulfurylase from plants. *Bioscience Reports*, *33*(4), e00053.
[41] Friedrich, M. W. (2002). Phylogenetic analysis reveals multiple lateral transfers of adenosine-5′-phosphosulphate reductase genes among sulphate-reducing microorganisms. *J Bacteriol*, *184*, 278–289.

[42] Fritz, G., Roth, A., Schiffer, A., et al. (2002). Structure of adenylylsulfate reductase from the hyperthermophilic *Archaeoglobus fulgidus* at 1.6-A resolution. *Proc. Natl. Acad. Sci. USA*, 99, 1836–1841.

[43] Kushkevych, I. V. (2014). Activity and kinetic properties of adenosine 5′-phosphosulfate reductase in the intestinal sulfate-reducing bacteria. *Microbiol & Biotechnol*, 2(26), 54–63.

[44] Kushkevych, I. V. & Fafula, R. V. (2014). Dissimilatory sulfite reductase in cell-free extracts of intestinal sulfate-reducing bacteria. *Studia Biologica*, 8(2), 101–112.

[45] Parey, K., Fritz, G., Ermler, U. & Kroneck, P. M. H. (2013). Conserving energy with sulfate around 100°C − structure and mechanism of key metal enzymes in hyperthermophilic *Archaeoglobus fulgidus*. *Metallomics*, 5, 302–317.

[46] Forzi, L., Koch, J., Guss, A. M., et al. (2005). Assignment of the 4Fe-4S clusters of ech hydrogenase from Methanosarcina barkeria to individual subunits via the characterization of site-directed mutants. *FEBS J*, 272, 4741–4753.

[47] Frederiksen, T. M. & Finster, K. (2003). Sulfite-oxido-reductase is involved in the oxidation of sulfite in *Desulfocapsa sulfoexigens* during disproportionation of thiosulphate and elemental sulfur. *Biodegradation*, 14, 189–198.

[48] Fritz, G., Buchert, T. & Kroneck, P. M. H. (2002). The Function of the [4Fe-4S] clusters and FAD in bacterial and archaeal adenylylsulfate reductases. *J. Biol. Chem*, 277, 26066–26073.

[49] Postgate, J. R. (1984). *The sulfate-reducing bakteria*. Cambridge University Press, Cambridge, 199 p.

[50] Rabus, R., Hansen, T. & Widdel, F. (2000). Dissimilatory Sulfate- and Sulfur-Reducing Prokaryotes//Dworkin M. et al. *The Prokaryotes. An Evolving Electronic Resource for the Microbiological Community*, 3rd edition. New York: Springer-Verlag.

[51] Broco, M., Rousset, M., Oliveira, S. & Rodrigues-Pousada, C. (2005). Deletion of flavoredoxin gene in *Desulfovibrio gigas* reveals its participation in thiosulphate reduction. *FEBS Lett*, 579, 4803–4807.

[52] Boronat, A., Britton, P., Jones-Mortimer, M. C., Kornberg, H. L., Lee, L. G., Murfitt, D. & Parra, F. (1984). Location on the Escherichia coli genome of a gene specifying O-acetylserine-(thiol)lyase. *J Gen Microbiol*, *130*, 673–685.

[53] Kushkevych, I. V. (2015). Molecular cloning *CysK* gene from *Escherichia coli* genome, transferring in the intestinal sulfate-reducing bacteria and the expression analysis of O-acetylserine-(thiol)lyase. *Microbes and Health*, *4*(1), 19–24.

[54] Kushkevych, I. V. & Antonyak, H. L. (2014). Activity of periplasmic hydrogenase of the intestinal sulfate-reducing bacteria. *The Animal Biology Journal*, *16*(2), 35–41.

[55] Odom, J. M. & Peck, H. D. (1984). Hydrogenase, electron-transfer proteins, and energy coupling in the sulphate-reducing bacteria *Desulfovibrio*. *Annu Rev Microbiol*, *38*, 551–592.

[56] Pohorelic, B. K., Voordouw, J. K., Lojou, E., et al. (2002). Effects of deletion of genes encoding Fe-only hydrogenase of *Desulfovibrio vulgaris* Hildenborough on hydrogen and lactate metabolism. *J Bacteriol*, *184*, 679–686.

[57] Goenka, A., Voordouw, J. K., Lubitz, W., et al. (2005). Construction of a NiFe-hydrogenase deletion mutant of *Desulfovibrio vulgaris* Hildenborough. *Biochem Soc Trans*, *33*, 59–60.

[58] Hedderich, R. (2004). Energy-converting NiFe hydrogenases from archaea and extremophiles: ancestors of complex I. *J Bioenerg Biomembr*, *36*, 65–75.

[59] Sapra, R., Bagramyan, K. & Adams, M. W. (2003). A simple energy-conserving system: proton reduction coupled to proton translocation. *Proc Natl Acad Sci USA*, *100*, 7545–7550.

[60] Černý, M., Vítězová, M., Vítěz, T., Bartoš, M. & Kushkevych, I. (2018). Variation in the distribution of hydrogen producers from the clostridiales order in biogas reactors depending on different input substrates. *Energies*, *11*(12), 3270.

[61] Kushkevych, I., Vítězová, M., Kos, J., et al. (2018). Effect of selected 8-hydroxyquinoline-2-carboxanilides on viability and sulfate metabolism of *Desulfovibrio piger*. *J App Biomed*, *16*, 241–246.

[62] Kushkevych, I., Kováč, J., Vítězová, M., et al. (2018). The diversity of sulfate-reducing bacteria in the seven bioreactors. *Archives of Microbiology*, *200*, 945–950.

[63] Gibson, G. R., Macfarlane, S. & Macfarlane, G. T. (1993). Metabolic interactions involving sulphate-reducing and methanogenic bacteria in the human large intestine. *FEMS Microbiol Ecol*, *12*, 117–125.

[64] Kushkevych, I., Vítězová, M., Vítěz, T., et al. (2017). Production of biogas: relationship between methanogenic and sulfate-reducing microorganisms. *Open Life Sciences*, *12*, 82–91.

[65] Brenner, D. J., Krieg, N. R., Staley, J. T. & Garrity, G. M. (2005). *Bergey's manual of Systematic Bacteriology. The Proteobacteria, Part C: The Alpha-, Beta-, Delta-, and Epsilonproteobacteria.* Second Edition. Printed in the USA, 1388 p.

[66] Moore, W. E., Johnson, J. L. & Holdeman, L. V. (1976). Emendation of *Bacteroidaceae* and *Butyrivibrio* and descriptions of *Desulfomonas* gen. nov. and ten new species of the genera *Desulfomonas, Butyrivibrio, Eubacterium, Clostridium* and *Ruminococcus*. *Int J Syst Bact*, *26*, 238–252.

[67] Loubinoux, J., Valente, F. M., Pereira, I. A., Costa, A., Grimont, P. A. & Le Faou, A. E. (2002). Reclassification of the only species of the genus *Desulfomonas*, *Desulfomonas pigra*, as *Desulfovibrio piger* comb. nov. *Int J Syst and Evol Microbiol*, *52*(4), 1305–1308.

[68] Kushkevych, I. V. (2013). Identification of sulfate-reducing bacteria strains of human large intestine. *Studia Biologica*, *7*(3), 115–124.

[69] Kushkevych, I. V., Bartos, M. & Bartosova, L. (2014). Sequence analysis of the 16S rRNA gene of sulfate-reducing bacteria isolated from human intestine. *Int J Curr Microbiol Appl Sci*, *3*(2), 239–248.

[70] Jobin, C. (2013). Colorectal cancer: looking for answers in the microbiota. *Cancer discovery*, *3*(4), 384–387.

[71] Loubinoux, J., Bronowicki, J. P., Pereira, I. A., Mougenel, J. L., Le Faou, A. E. (2002). Sulfate-reducing bacteria in human feces and their association with inflammatory bowel diseases. *FEMS microbiology ecology*, *40*(2), 107–112.

[72] Loubinoux, J., Bisson-Boutelliez, C., Miller, N. & Le Faou, A. E. (2002). Isolation of the provisionally named *Desulfovibrio fairfieldensis* from human periodontal pockets. *Oral Microbiol Immunol*, *17*, 321–323.

[73] Loubinoux, J., Jaulhac, B., Piemont, Y., Monteil, H., Le Faou, A. E. (2003). Isolation of sulfate-reducing bacteria from human thoracoabdominal pus. *J Clin Microbiol*, *41*(3), 1304–1306.

[74] Loubinoux, J., Mory, F., Pereira, I. A., Le Faou, A. E. (2000). Bacteremia caused by a strain of *Desulfovibrio* related to the provisionally named *Desulfovibrio fairfieldensis*. *J Clin Microbiol*, *38*, 931–934.

[75] Langendijk, P. S., Kulik, E. M., Sandmeier, H., Meyer, J., van der Hoeven, J. S. (2001). Isolation of *Desulfomicrobium orale* sp. nov. and *Desulfovibrio* strain NY682, oral sulfate-reducing bacteria involved in human periodontal disease. *J Syst Evol Microbiol*, *51*(3), 1035–1044.

[76] Verstreken, I., Laleman, W., Wauters, G., Verhaegen, J. (2012). *Desulfovibrio desulfuricans* bacteremia in an immunocompromised host with a liver graft and ulcerative colitis. *J Clin Microbiol*, *50*(1), 199–201.

[77] Goldstein, E. J. C., Citron, D. M., Peraino, V. A., Cross, S. A. (2003). *Desulfovibrio desulfuricans* bacteremia and review of human *Desulfovibrio* infections. *J Clin Microbiol*, *41*, 2752–2754.

[78] Tee, W., Dyall-Smith, M., Woods, W. & Eisen, D. (1996). Probable New Species of *Desulfovibrio* Isolated from a Pyogenic Liver Abscess. *J Clin Microbiol*, *34*(7), 1760–1764.

[79] McDougall, R., Robson, J., Paterson, D. & Tee, W. (1997). Bacteremia Caused by a Recently Described Novel *Desulfovibrio* Species. *J Clin Microbiol*, *35*(7), 1805–1808.

[80] Macfarlane, S., Hopkins, M. J., Macfarlane, G. T. (2000). Bacterial growth and metabolism on surfaces in the large intestine. *Microb Ecol Health Dis*, *2*, 64–72.

[81] Macfarlane, S. & Dillon, J. F. (2007). Microbial biofilms in the human gastrointestinal tract. *J Appl Microbiol*, *102*, 1187–1196.

[82] Zinkevich, V. V. & Beech, I. B. (2000). Screening of sulfate-reducing bacteria in colonoscopy samples from healthy and colitic human gut mucosa. *FEMS Microbiol Ecol*, *34*, 147–155.

[83] Probert, H. M. & Gibson, G. R. (2002). Bacterial biofilms in the human gastrointestinal tract. *Curr Iss Intest Microbiol*, *3*(2), 23–27.

[84] Fite, A., Macfarlane, G. T., Cummings, J. H., Hopkins, M. J., Kong, S. C., Furrie, E., Macfarlane, S. (2004). Identification and quantitation of mucosal and faecal desulfovibrios using real time polymerase chain reaction. *Gut*, *53*(4), 523–529.

[85] Gibson, G. R., Macfarlane, G. T. & Cummings, J. H. (1988). Occurrence of sulphate-reducing bacteria in human faeces and the relationship of dissimilatory sulphate reduction to methanogenesis in the large gut. *J Appl Bacteriol*, *65*, 103–111.

[86] Huovinen, J. A. & Gustaffson, B. E. (1967). Inorganic sulphate, sulphite and sulphide as sulphur donors in the biosynthesis of sulphur amino acids in germ-free and conventional rats. *Biochim Biophys Acta*, *136*, 441–447.

[87] Gibson, G. R., Cummings, J. H. & Macfarlane, G. T. (1988). Use of a three stage continuous culture system to study the effect of mucin on dissimilatory sulfate reduction and methanogenesis by mixed populations of human gut bacteria. *Appl Environ Microbiol*, *54*, 2750–2755.

[88] Perse, M. & Cerar, A. (2012). Dextran Sodium Sulphate Colitis Mouse Model: Traps and Tricks. *J Biomed and Biotech*, article ID 718617, 1–13.

[89] Low, D., Nguyen, D. D. & Mizoguchi, E. (2013). Animal models of ulcerative colitis and their application in drug research. *Drug Design, Development and Therapy*, *7*, 1341–1357.

[90] Zheng, L., Gao, Z. Q., Wang, S. X. (2000). A chronic ulcerative colitis model in rats. *World J Gastroenterol*, *6*(1), 150–152.

[91] Nell, S., Suerbaum, S., Josenhans, C. (2010). The impact of the microbiota on the pathogenesis of IBD: lessons from mouse infection models. *Nat Rev Microbiol*, *8*(8), 564–577.

[92] Barnett, M. & Fraser, A. (2011). Animal Models of Colitis: Lessons Learned, and Their Relevance to the Clinic. *Ulcerative Colitis*, 161–178.

[93] Sekirov, I., Russell, S. L., Antunes, L. C. M. & Finlay, B. B. (2010). Gut Microbiota in Health and Disease. *Physiol Rev*, *90*, 859–904.

[94] Kushkevych, I. V. (2014). Etiological role of sulfate-reducing bacteria in the development of inflammatory bowel diseases and ulcerative colitis. *Am J Infect Dis Microbiol*, *2*, 63–73.

[95] Kováč, J. & Kushkevych, I. (2017). New modification of cultivation medium for isolation and growth of intestinal sulfate-reducing bacteria. *Proceeding of Intern. PhD Stud Conf. MendelNet*, 702–707.

[96] Levine, J., Ellis, C. J., Furne, J. K., Springfield, J., Levitt, M. D. (1998). Fecal Hydrogen Sulfide Production in Ulcerative Colitis. *The Am J Gastroenterol*, *93*(1), 83–87.

[97] Ohge, H., Furne, J. K., Springfield, J., Sueda, T., Madoff, R. D., Levitt, M. D. (2003). The effect of antibiotics and bismuth on fecal hydrogen sulfide and sulfate-reducing bacteria in the rat. *FEMS Microbiol Lett*, *228*, 137–142.

[98] Levitt, M. D., Springfield, J., Furne, J., Koenig, T., Suarez, F. (2002). Physiology of sulfide in the rat colon: use of bismuth to assess colonic sulfide production. *J Appl Physiol*, *92*, 1655–1660.

[99] Levitt, M. D., Furne, J., Springfield, J., Suarez, F. & Demaster, E. (1999). Detoxification of hydrogen sulfide and methanethiol in the cecal mucosa. *J Clin Invest*, *104*, 1107–1114.

[100] Beauchamp, R. O., Bus, J. S., Popp, J. A., Boreiko, C. J., Andjelkovich, D. A. (1984). A critical review of the literature on hydrogen sulfide toxicity. *Crit Rev Toxicol*, *13*, 25–97.

[101] Suarez, F. L., Furne, J., Springfield, J., Levitt, M. D. (1998). Production and elimination of sulfur-containing gases in the rat colon. *Am J Physiol*, *274*, G727–G733.

[102] Chapman, M. A. S., Grahn, M. F., Boyle, M. A., et al. (1994). Butyrate oxidation is impaired in the colonic mucosa of sufferers of quiescent ulcerative colitis. *Gut*, *35*, 73–76.

[103] Roediger, W. E. W., Duncan, A., Kapaniris, O., Millard, S. (1993). Reducing sulfur compounds of colon impair colonocyte nutrition: implications for ulcerative colitis. *Gastroenterol, 104*, 802–809.
[104] Roediger, W. E. W., Duncan, A., Kapaniris, O., et al. (1993). Sulphide impairment of substrate oxidation in rat colonocytes: A biochemical basis for ulcerative colitis? *Clin Sci, 85*, 623–627.
[105] Roediger, W. E. W. & Nance, S. (1986). Metabolic induction of experimental ulcerative colitis by inhibition of fatty acid oxidation. *Br J Exp Pathol, 67*, 773–782.
[106] Sax, N. I. (1984). Dangerous properties of industrial materials. *Van Nostrand Reinhold Company*, New York.
[107] Vogt, J. A. & Wolever, T. M. S. (2003). Fecal Acetate Is Inversely Related to Acetate Absorption from the Human Rectum and Distal Colon. *J Nutr, 133*(10), 3145–3148.
[108] Walmsey, R. S., Anthony, A., Slim, R., et al. (1998). Absence of *Escherichia coli*, *Listeria moncytogenes*, and *Klebsiella pneumonae* antigens within inflammatory bowel disease tissues. *J Clin Pathol, 51*, 657–661.
[109] Kallinowski, F., Wassmer, A., Hofmann, M. A., et al. (1998). Prevalence of enteropathogenic bacteria in surgically treated chronic inflammatory bowel disease. *Hepatogastroenterol, 45*, 1552–1558.
[110] Campieri, M. & Gionchetti, P. (2001). Bacteria as the cause of ulcerative colitis. *Gut, 48*, 132–135.
[111] Burke, D. A. & Axon, A. T. R. (1988). Adhesive *Escherichia coli* in inflammatory bowel disease and infective diarrhea. *BMJ, 297*, 102–104.
[112] Burke, D. A. & Axon, A. T. R. (1987). Ulcerative colitis and *Escherichia coli* with adhesive properties. *J Clin Pathol, 40*, 782–786.
[113] Schultsz, C., Moussa, M., van Ketel, R., et al. (1997). Frequency of pathogenic and enteroadherent *Escherichia coli* in patients with inflammatory bowel disease and controls. *J Clin Pathol, 50*, 573–579.

[114] Von Wulffen, H., Rüssmann, H., Karch, H., et al. (1989). Verocytoxin-Producing *Escherichia coli* O2:H5 isolated from patients with ulcerative colitis. *Lancet, 1*, 1449–1450.

[115] Schultsz, C., van den Berg, F. M., Ten Kate, F. W., et al. (1999). The intestinal mucus layer from patients with inflammatory bowel disease harbours numbers of bacteria compared with controls. *Gastroenterol, 117*, 1089–1097.

[116] Onderdonk, A. B., Bronson, R. & Cisneros, R. (1987). Comparison of bacteroides vulgatus strains in the enhancement of experimental ulcerative colitis. *Infect Immun, 55*, 835–836.

[117] Rath, H. C., Ikeda, J. S., Linde, H. J., et al. (1999). Varying caecal bacterial loads influences colitis and gastritis in HLA-B27 transgenic rats. *Gastroenterol, 116*, 310–319.

[118] Ehrhardt, R. O., Lúdvíksson, B. R., Gray, B., et al. (1997). Induction and prevention of colonic inflammation in IL-2-deficient mice. *J Immunology, 158*, 566–573.

[119] Kuhn, R., Lohler, J., Rennick, D., et al. (1993). Interleukin-10-deficient mice develop chronic enterocolitis. *Cell, 75*, 263–274.

[120] Fite, A., Macfarlane, S., Furrie, E., et al. (2013). Longitudinal Analyses of Gut Mucosal Microbiotas in Ulcerative Colitis in Relation to Patient Age and Disease Severity and Duration. *J Clin Microbiol, 51*(3), 849–856.

[121] Kushkevych, I., Kollar, P., Suchy, P., et al. (2015). Activity of selected salicylamides against intestinal sulfate-reducing bacteria. *Neuroendocrinol Lett, 36*, 106–113.

[122] Kushkevych, I., Kollar, P., Ferreira, A. L., et al. (2016). Antimicrobial effect of salicylamide derivatives against intestinal sulfate-reducing bacteria. *J Appl Biomed, 14*, 125–130.

[123] Kushkevych, I., Kos, J., Kollar, P., et al. (2018). Activity of ring-substituted 8-hydroxyquinoline-2-carboxanilides against intestinal sulfate-reducing bacteria *Desulfovibrio piger*. *Med Chem Research, 27*, 278–284.

In: Colitis: Causes, Diagnosis and Treatment   ISBN: 978-1-53616-631-6
Editor: Soren Garcia   © 2019 Nova Science Publishers, Inc.

Chapter 3

HELMINTH THERAPY: A PROMISING BIOTHERAPEUTIC APPROACH FOR AUTOIMMUNE COLITIS

Kalyan Goswami[1,], MD, Vishal Khatri[2], PhD, Nitin Amdare[3], PhD, Namdev Togre[4], PhD and Priyanka Bhoj[5], PhD*

[1]Department of Biochemistry,
All India Institute of Medical Sciences, Kalyani, India
[2]Department of Biomedical Sciences,
University of Illinois College of Medicine, Rockford, IL, US
[3]Department of Microbiology and Immunology,
Albert Einstein College of Medicine, Montefiore, NY, US
[4]Department of Hepatitis, National Institute of Virology, Pune, India
[5]Department of Biochemistry,
Mahatma Gandhi Institute of Medical Sciences, Sevagram, India

---

[*] Corresponding Author's E-mail: goswamikln@gmail.com.

ABSTRACT

Of late, the incidence of autoimmune colitis both in adults and children has been progressively increasing globally. The efficacy of conventional therapeutic measures is questionably limited due to short-term immunosuppressive effect along with possible serious side effects. Evidence from epidemiological studies has demonstrated an inverse relationship between the occurrence of parasitic diseases and various autoimmune pathologies. Co-evolution of parasitic nematodes with humans possibly led to a positive selection pressure favoring a more tolerogenic immune response as an effective strategy of immune-evasion favoring long-term patency of parasitism. These immunomodulatory strategies have provided a significant cue for an alternative therapeutic approach. As proof of this premise, recent evidence has established a platform for the emergence of helminth-therapy as a promising alternative bio-therapeutics for colitis and other immune-mediated disorders. Studies in experimental models of colitis have shown that live/attenuated worms or their eggs or the soluble and/or excretory-secretory products of helminths have definitive therapeutic potential. Several clinical trials have also been conducted in colitis patients aiming to replicate the success of such experimental studies. However, utilization of live/attenuated worms or the crude products derived from them can cause serious complications with obvious ethical concerns, hence rendering these attempts controversial. Therefore, it seems more rational to explore and exploit specific immunomodulatory proteins from parasites having a more selective effect against colitis. Outcomes from the experimental studies that identified and demonstrated the efficacy of the use of certain recombinant parasitic proteins against ulcerative colitis have opened a new vista for developing helminth derived biotherapeutics against colitis. There is a definitive need to focus on this aspect for a better insight to utilize this novel therapeutic venture effectively and safely to resolve a very socially relevant health problem of recent times.

Keywords: Helminth therapy, recombinant proteins, ulcerative colitis, inflammatory bowel disease

1. THE ROLE OF NATURAL SELECTION PRESSURE OF NEMATODE INFECTION ON OUR IMMUNOME AND ITS CONSEQUENCE AS PER HYGIENE HYPOTHESIS

During the past four decades, there has been an exponential rise in the incidence of immunological disorders such as autoimmunity, allergy, and inflammatory disorders in economically developed societies, with a similar epidemiological pattern emerging in modernized areas of developing countries [1]. Evolving lifestyles with increasing sedentary habits along with altered dietary practices due to growing industrialization have contributed to the rapid transition towards autoimmune and/or chronic inflammatory disorders in epidemic proportion in modern societies. Moreover, genetic predisposition is the major underlying factor in the development of aberrant inflammatory responses [2-4]. Therefore, the emergence of many inflammatory disorders is apparently due to the interaction between evolutionarily selected genetic traits and environmental stimuli. Although such immunological patterns have been observed in the western world, lately the developing world has been exhibiting a similar trend.

Helminths are extraordinarily successful multicellular parasites due to their ability to modulate the host immune response, affecting around a quarter of the world's population [5]. Helminths have developed a wide range of strategies to manipulate the host immune system to survive and complete their reproductive cycles successfully and hence might be considered as a key evolutionary and ecological determinant of the homeostatic set point of the immune system of their hosts [6, 7]. Aiming to survive along with immuno-competent hosts, helminth parasites aim for the compensatory modification of the immune response through possible control over the expression of favourable molecules that disarm host immunity. This suggests that exposure to parasites has imposed strong evolutionary selective pressures on host immune associated genomes, now commonly known as '**immunomes**'. This underscores the fact that advantageous mutations in genes that confer a immune-phenotype to survive exposure to pathogens without severe inflammatory effect have been positively selected during evolution, whereas those leading to severe immune responses affecting the host have undergone negative selection; the later genes were subsequently removed from the host genome [3, 8, 9]. Until the recent past, it was just a speculated hypothesis that helminths are the major pathogenic group exerting such key selective force driving the evolution of specific components of the immune system. Indeed, the mechanisms of parasite-driven selection have been based on a single locus, namely major histocompatibility complex (MHC) polymorphism because of evolutionary interplay between parasite derived proteins and MHC-encoded proteins within a host individual [9, 10]. MHC genes are implicated in the adaptive immune response by the presentation of parasite-derived antigens to T lymphocytes which allows for parasite-mediated selection as a major evolutionary force [11, 12]. Furthermore, extensively investigated Toll-like receptors (TLR) are the large gene family that encodes important components of the innate immune system from the begining of its development. They have been co-opted independently to play a role in immune functions against pathogens in multiple species [13]. Whilst the advent of genome-wide studies have shown that during co-evolution with their hosts, some parasites, helminths in particular, have captured disease-associated SNPs and genes like interleukins (ILs) from their host to produce certain molecules that are able to disarm the host immunity; this shows the signature of positive selection, at least partially, as the consequence of past selective events to combat infection [10, 14]. Therefore, it can be envisaged that the current human immunome is the evolutionary consequence of marked and prolonged genetic selective pressure exerted by infectious pathogens [15, 16].

Modern lifestyle, improved sanitation barrier and advances in medical technology in economically stable societies predictably diminished the exposure to pathogens reducing such selection pressure, with resultant aberrant immune function due to unopposed individual genetic make-up [17]. Therefore, predictably human genes that have been tuned to the constant pressure of exposure to infectious agents, according to the "hygiene hypothesis" got insufficient exposure to parasites in the modern settings. Therefore, such populace would tend to express an immune phenotype with increased susceptibility towards the development of range of immune-mediated diseases today, such as type 1 diabetes, arthritis, multiple sclerosis, and inflammatory bowel disease (IBD). Based on the evolutionary legacy of gene selection in response to infectious pathogens, a role for helminths in the hygiene hypothesis cannot be overemphasized [18-20]. Furthermore, the use of helminth parasites as natural inducers of immune responses in experimental settings has delivered novel insights into multiple facets of immune function. Further understanding of the immunological genomes or 'immunomes' is the major key to unlock the potential of helminth therapy for immunomodulation in the clinical set up. A spectrum of helminth derived immunomodulatory molecules have evolved from helminth-host interaction that are now beginning to be defined, heralding a molecular revolution in parasite immunology. Although helminth therapy may not be suitable for all patients, however with additional research, the possibility to identify genotypic cohort for therapeutic suitability will ensure a dramatic improvement of efficacy rates. Close monitoring for vital changes in the immune assocaited genome to occur over time with such therapeutic modality, a more refined and elegant use for helminths in the clinic could be considered.

2. THE IMPACT AND EXISTING SCENARIO WITH A WHOLE WORM OR CRUDE ANTIGENS AS THERAPEUTIC OPTIONS FOR COLITIS

2.1. Whole Worm Therapy

The development of several animal models that can replicate the immunological and histopathological features of IBD conditions as in human has enabled evaluation of new therapeutic strategies in the preclinical phase [21-23]. These models have been extensively used to test the effect of heminth therapy on Crohn's and associated colitis conditions.

Elliott et al. [24] first confirmed that reduced exposure to helminths is associated with the increased risk of intestinal inflammation. The mice with *Schistosoma mansoni* infection were prevented from developing trinitrobenzene sulfonic acid (TNBS)-induced colitis. In the preliminary study, conducted by Reardon et al. [25], preventive or therapeutic treatment with *Hymenolepis diminuta* larvae showed improvement in the ion transport mechanism in the colon thus ameliorating the severity of dextran sulfate sodium (DSS)-colitis. The preventive treatment with *Trichinella spiralis* and *T. papuae* larvae was found to be associated with augmented Th2 immune response which exerts a protective effect on the dinitrobenzene sulfonic acid (DNBS) and DSS-induced colitis, respectively [26, 27]. Preventive treatment of mice with *T. spiralis* larvae and *T. papuae* larvae resulted in the amelioration of DNBS and DSS-induced colitis respectively [26, 27]. The treatment with *H. polygyrus bakeri* larvae showed suppression of colitis in piroxicam treated IL-10-/- mice [28, 29]. Also, treatment with *H. polygyrus bakeri* larvae found to have both preventive and therapeutic effects on colitis in IL10-/- T cell transfer mouse model [30, 31]. Donskow-Lysoniewska et al. [32] showed that curative treatment with *H. polygyrus bakeri* larvae ameliorated the severity of DSS-induced colitis with significantly reduced macrophage infiltration as determined by measuring reduced levels of IL-1β, TNF-α, and IL-6 cytokines.

The infection with *S. mansoni cercariae* and eggs prevents the severity of TNBS-induced colitis [33-35]. However, no attenuation effect was observed on DSS-induced colitis [34, 36]. In another study, Zhao et al. [37] reported that the prior treatment with *S. japonicum* eggs leads to prevention of TNBS-induced colitis disease course. The treatment of DSS-induced colitis mice with *S. mansoni* larvae resulted in reduced disease severity with lower levels of Th1 and Th2 cytokines [35]. These studies signify the importance of several species of helminths having both preventive and curative potential in different experimental colitis model as summarized in Table 1.

Table 1. Experimental animal studies with whole worm therapy

Helminth	Colitis model	Outcome of the study	References
H. diminuta larvae	DSS colitis	Restores colonic ion transport. No histopathological changes.	[25]
T. spiralis larvae	DNBS colitis	Increased Th2 response. Attenuated colitis symptoms.	[26]
S. mansoni eggs	TNBS colitis	Decreased IFN-γ, increased IL-4 and IL-10 expression.	[36]
S. mansoni larvae	TNBS colitis	Attenuate colitis with increased splenic IL-4 and IL-2 expression levels.	[33]
H. polygyrus bakeri larvae	IL-10-/-colitis	Decreased IL-12, IFN-γ and increased Th2, Treg response.	[28]
H. diminuta larvae	DNBS colitis	Increased IL-4, IL-10 mRNA expression. Reduces disease severity.	[38]
H. polygyrus bakeri larvae	IL10-/- T cell transfer colitis	Reverses inflammation with the induction of regulatory CD8+ T cells which inhibit T cell proliferation.	[30]
S. mansoni larvae	DSS colitis	Prevent colitis with the induction of regulatory macrophages (F4/80+CD11b+CD11c-).	[34]
S. japonicum eggs	TNBS colitis	Balanced Th1/Th2 response, downregulation of TLR4 mRNA expression, protects from colitis.	[37]
S. mansoni larvae	DSS colitis	Decreased TNF-α, IL-2 and IL-4 mRNA expression.	[39]
H. polygyrus bakeri larvae	IL10-/- T cell transfer colitis	Confers protection from colitis with the induction of tolerogenic DCs.	[31]
H. polygyrus bakeri larvae	Antigen driven colitis	Decreased IFN-γ, Th17, induction of Foxp3+ Treg cells, increased IL-10 from non-T cells.	[40]

DSS: dextran sulfate sodium; DNBS: dinitrobenzene sulfonic acid; TNBS: trinitrobenzene sulfonic acid; IL10-/-: IL-10 deficient; IFN-γ: interferon-γ; IL: interleukin; Foxp3: fork head box p3; STAT4: signal transducer and activator of transcription 4; TLR4: toll-like receptor 4; TNF-α: tumor necrosis factor-α; Treg: regulatory T cells; DCs: Dendritic cells.

Based on the encouraging outcomes from the myriad animal studies, clinical trials in humans were initiated. Although such venture had faced critical challenges from ethical and societal viewpoints of using live helminths for human therapy. A list of the same are summarized below:

Table 2. Clinical studies using helminth therapy in IBD patients

Details of the study	Outcome of the study	References
Single-dose of 2500 *T. suis* ova The repeated dose of 2500 *T. suis* ova at 3-wk intervals	No adverse effects were observed. Single dose effect: Remission in 75% CD patients and relapses in 67% within 12 wk. Remission in 100% of UC patients, 33% showed relapse within 12 wk. Repeated dose effect: 100% CD and UC patients achieved remission.	[41]
Repeated doses of 2500 *T. suis* ova at 3-wk intervals for 24 wk to 29 CD patients	No adverse effects were observed Remission noticed on 72.4% of patients within 24 wk.	[42]
Repeated doses of 2500 *T. suis* ova or placebo at 2-wk intervals for 12 wk. to 54 UC patients	No side effects. Remission noticed on 43.3% of patients.	[43]
The single or repeated dose of 25-50 L3 larvae *of N. americanus* administered to 9 CD patients.	Some adverse effects were observed. Disease activity index improved 20 wk. and 45 wk. post-infection.	[44]
Single-dose of 500, 2500 or 7500 live eggs of *T. suis* administered to 36 CD patients	No adverse effects were observed. 25.9% of ova-treated CD patients. 33.3% of placebo-treated CD patients reported gastrointestinal disturbances. 33.3% placebo-treated patients, 44.4% (500), 0% (2500) and 33.3% (7500) ova treated patients experienced at least 1 gastrointestinal disturbance.	[45]

UC: Ulcerative colitis; CD: Crohn's disease.

2.2. Crude Antigen Therapy

Promising results obtained in both human and animal studies prompted to test the efficacy of whole worms in clinical evaluations [42]. However, logically next step is to ensure protection from the expected maladies which may occur due to the use of live parasites for the treatment. Helminth therapy (HT) in its present form as standard therapy for the treatment of colitis is expected to be quite a difficult proposition due to certain drawbacks and obvious ethical considerations [46].

It is well known that HT uses whole live/attenuated worms, eggs or their crude extracts and that has been proven in providing beneficial results in abrogating Crohn's and colitis disease as well as other immune-regulated disorders (allergy, asthma, multiple sclerosis, and diabetes). Though proved beneficial in most human clinical trials, the research gathered limited scientific and medical knowledge regarding 1) the side-effects these worms can cause, 2) the mode-of-action, 3) safety issues (worms can carry other parasites such as bacteria with them), 4) operational guidelines for the use of HT (in case of incorrect protocol what are the risks involved), 5) correlation of specific helminths with a particular disease for their optimal benefit, 6) unwanted exposure to normal individuals, and 7) no systematic availability of clinical data. That is why, it is not surprising the difficulty in convincing both physicians and patients to use HT irrespective of all the unresolved drawbacks of currently available colitis therapeutics. Altogether, despite HT holding great potential for biotherapeutics, this promising therapy will prevail only if the existing limitations are addressed.

As a possible solution to obviate the adversities of HT, helminth-derived immunomodulatory molecules that could reproduce therapeutic effects of live/attenuated worms or their crude extracts on colitis has gained preference. Helminths secrete hundreds of molecules to allow them to survive within a host. Eventually, these molecules begin to interact with the host immune system and create a survivable environment for the helminths.

Over these past several years researchers have worked extensively to ascertain the pharmacological potential of such molecules derived from helminths in treating colitis and other immunological disorders [18, 23, 47]. Therefore, recent studies have focused on the characterization of helminth-derived products (HDPs) having potential immunosuppressive activity as the major prerequisite [48-50]. Certain examples of the same has been enlisted in Table 3.

Ruyssers et al. [51] showed treatment with *Ancylostoma ceylanicum* excretory/secretory products (AcES) resulted in amelioration of TNBS colitis with a significant decrease in IFN-γ, IL-17 along with increased level of regulatory cytokines IL-10, TGF-β. Protein molecules derived from *S. mansoni* soluble larval or adult proteins (SmSWP/SWAP) have been found to have an ameliorating effect on the TNBS and adaptive (CD4$^+$CD25$^-$CD62L$^+$T) T cell transfer model of colitis in mice [23, 51]. When used the antigen-based treatment strategy, the treatment with *T. spiralis* antigens was found to have a therapeutic effect on the DNBS-colitis with decreased myeloperoxidase activity and concomitant decrease in both IL-1β production and iNOS expression along with upregulation of IL-13 and TGF-β [52]. Also, the immunosuppressive activity of ES product from *H. diminuta* was found to be associated with the reduced TNF-α cytokine production and increased production of IL-10 and IL-4 [53]. Both curative and preventive treatment with *A. ceylanicum* ES products (AcES) and adult worm antigens (AcAw) have shown significant amelioration of DSS-induced colitis [54, 55].

In addition to IBD based evaluation of the therapeutic effect of helminth-derived products, many of these molecules are also being tested successfully in other inflammatory disease models. For example, the glycoproteins secreted by *S. mansoni* eggs omega-1 and IPSE/α-1 have shown to have a protective effect in type 1 diabetes model. Also, phosphorylcholine-containing glycoprotein (ES-62) secreted by *A. viteae*, was tested in rheumatoid arthritis model [57, 58].

Table 3. Animal studies with crude or extracted helminth proteins

Helminth	Colitis model	Outcome of the study	References
S. mansoni soluble egg antigen (SEA)	CD4$^+$CD25$^-$CD62$^+$ T cell transfer colitis	Attenuate colitis with decreased Th17 response, increased Th2 response.	[56]
S. mansoni worm adult proteins (SWAP)	CD4$^+$CD25$^-$CD62$^+$ T cell transfer colitis	Significant decrease in IFN-γ, Th17A RNA expression and augmented Th2 response confers protection.	[56]
A. ceylanicum (AcES)	DSS colitis	Protect from colitis with decreased Pro-inflammatory response.	[55]
A. ceylanicum adult worm crude extract (AcAw) and excretory-secretory proteins (AcES)	DSS colitis	Decreased Th1 response (IFN-γ, TNF-α), diminished Th17 response (IL-17).	[54]
H. diminuta high molecular mass (HdHMW)	DNBS colitis	Decreased TNF-α expression. Increased IL-4, IL-10 offers colitis protection.	[53]
T. spiralis antigen	DNBS colitis	Attenuate colitis with increased TGF-β expression and downregulated IL-1β and iNOS.	[52]
S. mansoni soluble worm proteins (SmSWP)	TNBS colitis	Protects from colitis. Downregulated IFN-γ, Th17 mRNA expression, increased Treg response.	[51]

DSS: dextran sulfate sodium; DNBS: dinitrobenzene sulfonic acid; TNBS: trinitrobenzene sulfonic acid; IFN-γ: interferon-γ; Th: T-helper; Treg: T-regulatory; TNF-α: tumor necrosis factor-α; Treg: regulatory T cells; CD: Cluster of differentiation.

3. RECOMBINANT PROTEINS AS THERAPEUTICS FOR COLITIS

Towards a further advancement of this parasitic protein based therapeutic tool, research has focused on recombinant technology to develop precise molecule of interest having specific immunomodulatory effect. As a method recombinant technology is more robust and amenable to provide high-throughput delivery with precision. Therefore this new-age technique has steered the present research to a new height.

The most important determinant of success for this approach lies in the apposite choice of the candidate protein which is endowed with precise immunomodulatory effect without much cross reactivity causing untoward impact. Therefore, it is of paramount importance to select such protein with the utmost care and then expose it to rugged research methods with stringent standards for validating its efficacy and safety.

Since helminth parasites remain in extracellular locale, the immune system depends upon exogenous pathways of antigen presentation. Hence for development of protective immune response against them, the foreign antigens must be processed by lysosomal proteinases such as aspartyl or cysteine proteinases within endosomal-lysosomal compartments of antigen presenting cells (APC) and such processed peptides must be presented by major histocompatibility complex (MHC class II) molecules expressed on the APCs. Therefore, the inhibition of these proteinases in the host can lead to drastic changes in antigen processing and prevent the generation of peptide-MHC-II complex formation. Consequently, that could lead to reduction in antigen presentation which in turn would be able to deteriorate protective immune response by the host. Many studies have reported in favor of this view by showing helminth parasite induced block of the antigen presentation pathway in the host's APC; especially filarial parasites such as *Brugia malayi* [59], *Litmosoides sigmodontis* [60], *Onchocerca volvulus* [61] displayed such effect. This body of evidence suggests that proteinase inhibitors are utilized by filarial parasites as immunomodulators to protect themselves.

Among proteinase inhibitors, cystatin belongs to cysteine proteinase-inhibitory proteins superfamily. Cysteine protease inhibitors (cystatins) are the first and most-studied immunomodulatory molecules secreted by helminths. *B. malayi* secretes cystatin which interferes with two classes of proteinases in MHC class II pathway, the papain like cathepsin B, L and S and the legumains-type asparagine endopeptidase. Immunomodulatory properties of filarial cystatin are attributed to the induction of hyporeactivity in T cells, modulation of production of cytokines and downregulation of essential co-stimulatory molecules on macrophages [61, 62]. In fact, cystatins participate in many vital immunological processes such as antigen processing and presentation, migration of immune cells, activation of toll-like receptors and cytokines secretion [63-66]. Cystatins also alternatively activate IL-10 producing macrophages to be recruited in various effector arms of the immune system [18, 67]. All these properties of cystatin makes it a molecule of interest for the treatment of colitis.

Treatment with *Acanthocheilonema viteae* cystatin (AvCystatin) reduced the inflammatory index of the colon in DSS plus AvCystatin-treated mice by up to 54% [68]. This study emphasized the role of Th2-macrophages in the suppression of inflammatory conditions by cystatin. Adoptive transfer of AvCystatin-M regulatory (Mregs) cells had suppressed the pathology of DSS-colitis [67]. AvCystatin-Mregs are alternatively activated by the M2a/M2b phenotype and the activation of Mregs was independent of IL-10. A study has also utilized novel transgenic bacterium secreting AvCystatin that could potentially reduce DSS-induced colitis pathology in both mouse and piglets model, where it significantly reduced inflammatory score compared to the control [69]. More studies have highlighted the therapeutic efficacy of recombinant cystatins from *S. japonicum, Ascaris lumbricoides, Clonorchis sinensis* and *T. spiralis* [70-73]. Of late, our group has shown that recombinant cystatin from filarial *B. malayi* parasite has improved the clinico-pathologic condition of both acute and chronic DSS mediated colitis in mice [49, 74]. Filarial parasites are long-lived in their host and cystatin derived from them has been shown to be highly immunosuppressive in nature [61, 75-77].

Furthermore, similar evidence has been gathered with several other proteins like; 53-kDa protein (rTs-P53) of *T. spiralis*, rAs-MIF of *Anisakis simplex*; asparaginyl-tRNA synthase and abundant larval transcript (ALT-2) proteins from *B. malayi*, galectin-9 homolog (rTl-GAL) of *Toxascaris leonine*, P53 protein from *T. spiralis*, Calreticulin from *Taenia solium* and rSj16 from *S. japonicum* have attenuated DSS/TNBS/T cell-induced colitis in mice or rats [78-85]. Treatment with these proteins suppressed the colitis symptoms such as weight loss, hematochezia, colon damage, and mucosal edema. Involvement of T-regulatory cells (Tregs) and macrophages has been associated with the proposed rationale of the immunomodulatory mechanisms of these molecules.

Interestingly, Glutathione S-transferases (GSTs) secreted by the helminths are vital in reducing oxidative stress initiated by the host's immune system towards the invading parasite; which makes GSTs a great potential vaccine candidate against helminth infections. The 28-kDa Glutathione-S-transferase enzyme (P28GST) of *S. mansoni* has shown to reduce the detrimental effects of TNBS-induced colitis in rats [86]. The results were similar to parasite-infected group, which suggests that besides a full parasite infection, a single molecule can also significantly limit the colitis condition. P28GST-treated induced-colitis mice shown reduced levels of IL-1β, IFN-γ, TNF-α, and IL-17 and a skew towards Th2-immune response (increased expression of IL-5, IL-10, and IL-13) in the colon. Eosinophils have been showed to be majorly involved in P28GST-mediated attenuation of colitis. Delivery of *S. haematobium* GST loaded PLGA-beads into TNBS-colitis mice yielded significant suppression of colitis related symptoms [87]. Results of a recent study reinforced that P28GST can relieve the symptoms in TNBS-colitis [88]. P28GST has successfully gone through phase 1 in clinical trials for safety and immunogenicity studies (NCT01512277) and phase 2 clinical trials in CD patients has been recently completed (NCT02281916).

Table 4. Animal studies with recombinant proteins from helminths

Recombinant molecule	Parasite	Colitis model	Outcome of the study	Reference
Cysteine protease inhibitors (Cystatins)	A. viteae	DSS-colitis	54% suppression of inflammatory index of the colon. Improved colon pathology. Role of IL-10 producing macrophages.	[68]
	A. viteae	DSS-colitis / Intestinal inflammation in pigs	Utilized genetically modified probiotic bacterium Escherichia coli Nissle 1917 to secrete AvCys in the gut. Decreased intestinal inflammation in mice and pigs.	[69]
Cysteine protease inhibitors (Cystatins)	A. viteae	DSS-colitis	Adoptive transfer of Mregs to reduce acute intestinal inflammation. 100% recovery from body weight loss. Decreased colon damage. Significant decrease in the histopathological score and MPO activity in the colon.	[67]
	B. malayi	DSS-colitis	Significant reduction in weight loss and DAI. Reduced colon damage and cellular infiltration. Improved pathology of the colon.	[74]
		DSS-chronic colitis	Reduction in weight loss. Improved clinic-pathologic condition of chronic colitis.	[49]
	S. japonicum	TNBS-colitis	No improvement in weight loss and DAI. Reduced microscopic score and MPO activity of the colon.	[70]
	A. lumbricoides	DSS- colitis	Attenuation of the disease condition. Significant reduction in DAI, MPO activity and histopathological damage of colon.	[71]

Table 4. (Continued)

Recombinant molecule	Parasite	Colitis model	Outcome of the study	Reference
	C. sinensis	DSS-colitis	Curative treatment lead to the amelioration of colitis condition. Decreased TNF-α. Role of IL-10 producing macrophages.	[72]
Cysteine protease inhibitors (Cystatins)	T. spiralis	TNBS-colitis	Reduced DAI, MPO activity, and colon pathology. Increased IL-4 in the colon.	[73]
Recombinant larvae 53 kDa glycoprotein (TsP53)	T. spiralis	TNBS-colitis	Reduced colitis condition. Lower serum levels of TNF-α, IFN-γ Increased levels of Arg-1, Fizz1, IL-10, and TGF-β.	[78]
Macrophage migratory inhibitory factor (MIF) homolog	A. simplex	DSS-colitis	Reduced DAI, weight loss and colitis pathology. TLR-2 mediated suppression of colitis. Increased levels of IL-10 and TGF-β.	[79]
Abundant larval transcript protein	B. malayi	DSS-colitis	Reduced DAI, weight loss and colitis pathology.	[80]
Asparaginyl-tRNA synthase		T-cell transfer model	Reduced colitis pathology.	[81]
Galectin-9	T. leonine	DSS-colitis	Reduced DAI, weight loss and colitis pathology. Increased levels of IL-10 and TGF-β.	[82]
28-kDa Glutathione S transferase	S. mansoni	TNBS-colitis	Reduced clinical signs and pathology of colitis. Reduction in colonic MPO. Increased levels of colonic IL-13 and IL-5.	[86]

Recombinant molecule	Parasite	Colitis model	Outcome of the study	Reference
28-kDa Glutathione S transferase	S. haematobium	TNBS-colitis	Eosinophil-dependent modulation of Th1-inflammatory condition. Subcutaneous treatment of GST loaded PLGA-beads reduced colitis condition. Reduced clinicopathologic symptoms of colitis. Decreased levels of TNF, IL-1β, and IL6. Decreased expression of T-bet, and ROR-γ. Induction of M2 macrophages.	[87] [88]
P53	T. spiralis	TNBS-colitis	Reduced expression of TNF-α, IFN-γ, IL-6 cytokines. Increased expression of IL-10 and TGF-β. Alternative activation of macrophages.	[83]
rSj16	S. japonicum	DSS-colitis	Attenuated clinical colitis symptoms. Role of peroxisome proliferator-activated receptor α in the colon.	[85]

DSS: dextran sulfate sodium; TNBS: trinitrobenzene sulfonic acid; DAI: disease activity score; MPO: myeloperoxidase activity; TNF-α: tumor necrosis factor-α; TGF-β: transforming growth factor-β; Treg: T-regulatory cells; IFN-γ: interferon-γ.

To summarize, based on the outcomes from experimental studies, specific molecules do have a definite edge over traditional HT in suppressing colitis. The future for helminth-derived biomolecules as therapeutics of colitis is bright. However, certain questions are to be answered before using them to clinics.

4. IMPACT OF HELMINTH THERAPY ON THE IMMUNE STATUS AND ITS POSSIBLE RATIONALE

The helminths have adopted remarkable abilities and sophisticated mechanisms which can modulate several immune regulatory pathways and counter the host inflammatory immune reactions for their own survival [50]. This unique property of helminths could render them highly effective at controlling inflammatory and autoimmune disorders, such as inflammatory bowel disease, diabetes, and asthma [50, 89, 90]. Several experimental studies and human trials emphasize the significance of HT on immune-mediated diseases through the activation of T regulatory cells, downregulation of toll-like receptors (TLRs), and expression of anti-inflammatory cytokines, such as TGF-β and IL-10 [4, 23, 71].

Initial studies emphasized helminth induced production of IL-4 secreting Th-2 cells that inhibit inflammatory Th 1 immune cell response. Inhibition of Th-2 function promoted both Th-1 cell differentiation and persistence of colitis in the mouse model, indicating the significance of helminth-induced Th-2 response in disease control. However, helminthic infections are also known to ameliorate Th-2 driven allergic reactions. This apparent paradoxical effect prompted researchers to explore additional mechanisms of helminth induced immune regulation independent of Th-2 cells and cytokines.

Several T-cell subsets aid-in disease amelioration. Adoptive transfer of Foxp3$^+$ T cells from the mesenteric lymph nodes (MLN-T cells) of *H. polygyrus bakeri*-infected mice into IL-10-/-colitic mouse model can abrogate established colitis, showing the significance of Foxp3$^+$ Tregs in colitis control [28]. In mouse colon, 20% of lamina propria CD4⁺ T cells are Foxp3⁺ Tregs and half of the Foxp3+ Tregs also express IL-10. The number of IL10 and/or TGFβ secreting Treg cells increases in the MLNs and the intestinal lining during helminthic infection that inhibit Th-1 responses and colitis in animal models [91]. IL-10 plays an important role in mucosal protection as IL-10-/- transgenic mice develop severe Th-1 type colitis. *H. polygyrus* also enhance a small proportion of CD8⁺Tregs in the intestine that inhibits splenic T cell proliferation in an MHC-I dependent manner through cell-cell contact. These cells may be important for colitis protection, and do not require the involvement of IL-10 and TGF-β.

It is not fully elucidated how the several regulatory T cells get involved in colitis control. One possible mechanism is through the production of regulatory cytokines that inhibit effector cytokine production. As regulatory cytokine, IL-10 inhibits the production of several pro-inflammatory cytokines viz. TNF-α and IL-12 and tends to block the activity of inflammatory-macrophage and dendritic cells. *S. mansoni* and *H. polygyrus bakeri* protect mice from TNBS-induced colitis by stimulating IL-10 and TGF-β production which reduces IFN-γ production from Th-1 type effector T cells and limits IL-12 p40 release. IL-12 p40 is a potent IL-12 agonist and is a critical pathogenic factor in intestinal inflammation [92]. TGF-β is another immunomodulatory cytokine in inflammatory colitis having a stimulatory effect on the production of regulatory T cells, and the suppression of dendritic cells and macrophages. Interestingly, TGF-β orthologs have been characterized in several helminths including *A. caninum, B. malayi, F. hepatica, H. polygyrus*, and *Schistosoma genus*. IL-17 secreting Th17 cells play a major role in the persistence of colitis. *H. polygyrus bakeri* promotes IL-4 and IL-10 production that impedes IL-17 secretion; moreover, IL-4 plays an important role in IL-17 regulation. Owing to Th-2 promoting and concomitant Th-1 suppressing immune responses, coupled with the alternative activation of macrophages that are implicated in wound healing mediated by IL-4, it exerts robust anti-colitic impact. This interleukin also promotes production and secretion of mucus, which protects the gut from irritants.

Helminths also offer protection from IBD through macrophage and dendritic cells-dependent pathways. In the host immune system, lysosomal cysteine proteases play an important role in exogenous antigen processing and presentation on macrophages and dendritic cells. However, helminth cystatin, a cysteine protease inhibitor, blocks the protease inhibitors from host myeloid cells. The *B. malayi* cystatin, CPI-2 inhibit lysosomal asparaginyl endopeptidase (AEP) and cathepsins leading to the blockade of MHC-class II-restricted antigen processing [93]. Onchocystatin from *Onchocerca volvulus* reduces MHC-II and CD86 expression (costimulatory signals required for T cell activation) with the induction of IL-10 expression in human monocytes in vitro. These results are confirmed with *in vivo* mouse models, as *A. viteae* cystatin results in increased expression of IL-10 in macrophages conferring protection against both airway allergy and colitis [94]. Other helminth cystatins from *S. japonicum, A. lumbricoides, and C. sinensis* also have immunomodulatory properties which lead to amelioration of colitis *in vivo* [70-72], the physiological target of these proteins are yet to be identified. Helminthic infections stimulate the host to produce IL-10 and Th2 cytokines such as IL-4 and IL-5. These cytokines "alternatively" activate macrophages (AAMs), which induce production of TGF-β, IL-10, and other immune-modulatory factors.

Cellular immunotherapy is emerging as a novel stratagem of helminth based therapy for colitis. Adoptive transfer of *H. diminuta* somatic extract-treated dendritic cells (HD-DCs) significantly reduced the severity of DNBS-induced colitis through IL-4Rα signaling. Administration of IL-4Rα$^{+/+}$ HD-DCs induced IL-4 production in recipient splenic T-cells. Recipient IL-4 is the source for IL-4Rα activation on HD-DCs. IL-4Rα-activated HD-DCs produce IL-10 *in vivo* and drive the further synthesis of IL-4 and IL-10 in recipient mice [95]. Significance of IL-4Rα-IL-4 signaling can be further attested by the production of CD4$^+$T cells and CD19$^+$B cells as sources of IL-4 in HD-DC recipient colitic mice [96]. Adaptive transfer of splenic CD19$^+$B cells, which are the source of TGFβ, from mice infected previously with *H. diminuta* (HD-CD19+ B cells) significantly reduced the severity of oxazolone, DNBS, and DSS- induced colitis. Mechanistic studies with RAG1$^{-/-}$ mice revealed no requirement of T and B cells in the recipient, as HD-CD19$^+$B cells inhibited colitis in this mouse model. However, depletion of macrophages in recipient colitic mice failed to show the anti-colitic effect of HD-CD19$^+$ B cells signifying involvement of macrophages. Adoptive transfer of *T. spiralis*-activated AAMs has also been shown to ameliorate colitic inflammation in murine models [97].

A schistosome enzymatic protein, the 28-kDa glutathione-S-transferase (P28GST) represents a new immuno-regulatory strategy against colitis. P28GST induced the increase in IL-13 and IL-5 cytokines, with significant infiltration of colonic lamina propria by eosinophils in the colitic rat as well as mouse models. Eosinophils are associated with a Th-2 immune profile. IL-13 (and possibly, IL-4) released by eosinophils activates IL-10 producing AAMs. Due to the high degree purity in P28GST production without any cross-reactivity with human GSTs (indicating safety in human use), it has undergone phase 1 clinical trials for safety and immunogenicity studies (NCT01512277) and is currently in a phase 2 trial in Crohn's disease (NCT02281916).

Interestingly, helminths produce some host cytokine orthologs and modulate innate cell response via molecular mimicry. For example, *B. malayi* macrophage migration inhibitory factor (MIF) mimics the activity of the host protein, with the release of TNF-α, IL-8 and endogenous MIF from monocytes. However, high levels of MIF actually block AP-1 dependent pro-inflammatory gene expression by binding to an intracellular co-activator of AP-1 transcription factor, Jab1. Also, in the presence of IL-4, *Bm*MIF induces alternatively activated macrophage stimualtion with the development of type-2 immune reactivity. Therefore, by secreting MIF at the site of infection, helminths also might induce further synthesis of endogenous host MIF, creating a systemic anti-inflammatory environment [98]. MIF from *Anisakis simplex* is anti-inflammatory, suppressing both allergy and colitis in mice [99].

Therefore, it may be concluded that helminths do not regulate intestinal inflammation through induction of only one cytokine or single regulatory circuit. They control several distinct, complex and interconnected pathways, mainly associated with innate immunity. Also, not all helminths use similar mechanisms for the host immunomodulation.

5. THE MAJOR LESSONS LEARNT FROM EXPERIMENTAL STUDIES, MERITS AND DEMERITS

The conventional therapies for colitis are non-specific with short-term immunosuppressive effects, expensive and require longer duration of therapy leading to lack of patient compliance. These therapies also increase risk of opportunistic infections and cancer development [100]. Presently, 5-aminosalicylates (5-ASA), anti-TNF-α (infiximab), mesalamine and corticosteroids are the most widely used therapeutics for the treatment of IBD. These treatment options have various side effects like nausea, headache, diarrhea, insomnia, osteoporosis, non-Hodgkins lymphoma and can increase the risk of hepatosplenic T cell lymphoma [101-104]. These drawbacks highlight the need for development of new therapeutic approaches for UC.

The potential of HT to treat autoimmune diseases has been demonstrated in animal models and many clinical trials. Humans being natural hosts to helminths, HT can be well tolerated by patients suffering from IBD. HT is without doubt a superior, less expensive and safer alternative to current therapies. Eventhough, HT can cause discomfort in some patients from clinical trials, the side-effects can never be life-threatning or detrimental compared to the current therapies. Although, outcomes from clinical trials suggest remission in IBD patients, results were less conclusive due to certin flaws in experimental design, requiring additional research.

Experimental studies using identified immunomodulatory molecules maintain the enthusiasm of bringing HT to clinics. Although limited, most of the experimental studies demonstrate that the beneficial effects of live worms or crude extracts could be translated in a better way by using the recombinant molecules in IBD. Results are awaited from the very first clinical trail using GST. It is imperative that, more extensive and well planned studies with these molecules be conducted and addressing unresolved issues before such therapy can be practiced in clinics.

- There should be a clear understanding of how these molecules work in colitis or any other inflammatory condition.
- Although recombinant biomedicines are probably the safest treatment options, any undesirable side-effects these molecules can cause in colitis patients, need to be identified.
- Following the drugs being waned off from the body, there can be a resurgence of the disease condition. A detailed knowledge of the strength and number of dosages to be administered to colitis or IBD patients is required. It is also important to ascertain whether these beneficial effects of drugs could be extended for a longer period of time.
- Insight into the effect these drugs may have on those already suffering from other disorders (cancer, HIV etc.) is also crucial.
- The best way to administer these drugs into a human is yet to be validated.
- The knowledge about whether these molecules are disease-specific or can act as broad spectrum immune modulator for all types of allergies and autoimmune disorders is imperative.

6. THE FUTURE PERSPECTIVE

As discussed above, to date most of the clinical trials are conducted with live helminths, which might be associated with the risk of parasite infestation, lack immunological specificity, and may lead to detrimental patho-physiological effects besides other ethical and societal issues. Therefore, treatment with purified helminth derived products is more desirable, which demands exploration of its therapeutic rationale and safety. Furthermore, these proteins can be recombinantly synthesized in large quantities at a relatively reasonable cost. With the aim of site-directed therapy and sustained immunomodulatory effect, these proteins can be delivered to affected inflammatory site using probiotic carriers with the ability to recombinantly synthesize and release desired immunomodulators.

The majority of clinical studies conducted to date were not properly controlled, comprised small sample sizes with a lack of standardized doses, and/or did not use human-tropic helminths. Forthcoming trials should address these limitations. Few research teams have evaluated the potential of recombinant proteins of human dwelling parasites in colitic mouse models, with significant disease ameliorating results. However, the detailed mechanism of action of these proteins with precise pharmacological targets needs to be explored in order to nudge this research towards a translational level.

Tremendous research in the current era of omics like genomics, proteomics, and metabolomics to develop insight into parasitic biology and its interaction with human immune system can foster the course of discovery of novel and potent helminth-derived immunomodulators. Undoubtedly, many potential helminth-derived bio-therapeutics will be explored to get an edge over the conventional therapeutics against colitis in the coming years.

REFERENCES

[1] Moroni, L., I. Bianchi, and A. Lleo. 2012. "Geoepidemiology, gender and autoimmune disease." *Autoimmun Rev* 11 (6-7):A386-92. doi: 10.1016/j.autrev.2011.11.012.

[2] Precechtelova, J., M. Borsanyiova, S. Sarmirova, and S. Bopegamage. 2014. "Type I diabetes mellitus: genetic factors and presumptive enteroviral etiology or protection." *J Pathog* 2014:738512. doi: 10.1155/2014/738512.

[3] Khan, A. R., and P. G. Fallon. 2013. "Helminth therapies: translating the unknown unknowns to known knowns." *Int J Parasitol* 43 (3-4):293-9. doi: 10.1016/j.ijpara.2012.12.002.

[4] Weinstock, J. V., and D. E. Elliott. 2014. "Helminth infections decrease host susceptibility to immune-mediated diseases." *J Immunol* 193 (7):3239-47. doi: 10.4049/jimmunol.1400927.

[5] Bethony, J., S. Brooker, M. Albonico, S. M. Geiger, A. Loukas, D. Diemert, and P. J. Hotez. 2006. "Soil-transmitted helminth infections: ascariasis, trichuriasis, and hookworm." *Lancet* 367 (9521):1521-32. doi: 10.1016/S0140-6736(06)68653-4.

[6] Jackson, J. A., I. M. Friberg, S. Little, and J. E. Bradley. 2009. "Review series on helminths, immune modulation and the hygiene hypothesis: immunity against helminths and immunological phenomena in modern human populations: coevolutionary legacies?" *Immunology* 126 (1):18-27. doi: 10.1111/j.1365-2567.2008.03010.x.

[7] King, I. L., and Y. Li. 2018. "Host-Parasite Interactions Promote Disease Tolerance to Intestinal Helminth Infection." *Front Immunol* 9:2128. doi: 10.3389/fimmu.2018.02128.

[8] Leonardi-Bee, J., D. Pritchard, and J. Britton. 2006. "Asthma and current intestinal parasite infection: systematic review and meta-analysis." *Am J Respir Crit Care Med* 174 (5):514-23. doi: 10.1164/rccm.200603-331OC.

[9] Sommer, S. 2005. "The importance of immune gene variability (MHC) in evolutionary ecology and conservation." *Front Zool* 2:16. doi: 10.1186/1742-9994-2-16.

[10] Spurgin, L. G., and D. S. Richardson. 2010. "How pathogens drive genetic diversity: MHC, mechanisms and misunderstandings." *Proc Biol Sci* 277 (1684):979-88. doi: 10.1098/rspb.2009.2084.

[11] Eizaguirre, C., T. L. Lenz, M. Kalbe, and M. Milinski. 2012. "Rapid and adaptive evolution of MHC genes under parasite selection in experimental vertebrate populations." *Nat Commun* 3:621. doi: 10.1038/ncomms1632.

[12] Prugnolle, F., A. Manica, M. Charpentier, J. F. Guegan, V. Guernier, and F. Balloux. 2005. "Pathogen-driven selection and worldwide HLA class I diversity." *Curr Biol* 15 (11):1022-7. doi: 10.1016/j.cub.2005.04.050.

[13] Kettenmann, H., U. K. Hanisch, M. Noda, and A. Verkhratsky. 2011. "Physiology of microglia." *Physiol Rev* 91 (2):461-553. doi: 10.1152/physrev.00011.2010.

[14] Fumagalli, M., U. Pozzoli, R. Cagliani, G. P. Comi, S. Riva, M. Clerici, N. Bresolin, and M. Sironi. 2009. "Parasites represent a major selective force for interleukin genes and shape the genetic predisposition to autoimmune conditions." *J Exp Med* 206 (6):1395-408. doi: 10.1084/jem.20082779.

[15] Maizels, R. M. 2005. "Infections and allergy - helminths, hygiene and host immune regulation." *Curr Opin Immunol* 17 (6):656-61. doi: 10.1016/j.coi.2005.09.001.

[16] Barreiro, L. B., and L. Quintana-Murci. 2010. "From evolutionary genetics to human immunology: how selection shapes host defence genes." *Nat Rev Genet* 11 (1):17-30. doi: 10.1038/nrg2698.

[17] Casanova, J. L., and L. Abel. 2005. "Inborn errors of immunity to infection: the rule rather than the exception." *J Exp Med* 202 (2):197-201. doi: 10.1084/jem.20050854.

[18] Maizels, R. M., H. H. Smits, and H. J. McSorley. 2018. "Modulation of Host Immunity by Helminths: The Expanding Repertoire of Parasite Effector Molecules." *Immunity* 49 (5):801-818. doi: 10.1016/j.immuni.2018.10.016.

[19] Okada, H., C. Kuhn, H. Feillet, and J. F. Bach. 2010. "The 'hygiene hypothesis' for autoimmune and allergic diseases: an update." *Clin Exp Immunol* 160 (1):1-9. doi: 10.1111/j.1365-2249.2010.04139.x.

[20] Yazdanbakhsh, M., P. G. Kremsner, and R. van Ree. 2002. "Allergy, parasites, and the hygiene hypothesis." *Science* 296 (5567):490-4. doi: 10.1126/science.296.5567.490.

[21] Wirtz, S., and M. F. Neurath. 2007. "Mouse models of inflammatory bowel disease." *Adv Drug Deliv Rev* 59 (11):1073-83. doi: 10.1016/j.addr.2007.07.003.

[22] Mizoguchi, A., and E. Mizoguchi. 2008. "Inflammatory bowel disease, past, present and future: lessons from animal models." *J Gastroenterol* 43 (1):1-17. doi: 10.1007/s00535-007-2111-3.

[23] Heylen, M., N. E. Ruyssers, E. M. Gielis, E. Vanhomwegen, P. A. Pelckmans, T. G. Moreels, J. G. De Man, and B. Y. De Winter. 2014. "Of worms, mice and man: an overview of experimental and clinical helminth-based therapy for inflammatory bowel disease." *Pharmacol Ther* 143 (2):153-67. doi: 10.1016/j.pharmthera.2014.02.011.

[24] Elliott, D. E., Jf Jr Urban, C. K. Argo, and J. V. Weinstock. 2000. "Does the failure to acquire helminthic parasites predispose to Crohn's disease?" *FASEB J* 14 (12):1848-55. doi: 10.1096/fj.99-0885hyp.

[25] Reardon, C., A. Sanchez, C. M. Hogaboam, and D. M. McKay. 2001. "Tapeworm infection reduces epithelial ion transport abnormalities in murine dextran sulfate sodium-induced colitis." *Infect Immun* 69 (7):4417-23. doi: 10.1128/IAI.69.7.4417-4423.2001.

[26] Khan, W. I., P. A. Blennerhasset, A. K. Varghese, S. K. Chowdhury, P. Omsted, Y. Deng, and S. M. Collins. 2002. "Intestinal nematode infection ameliorates experimental colitis in mice." *Infect Immun* 70 (11):5931-7. doi: 10.1128/iai.70.11.5931-5937.2002.

[27] Adisakwattana, P., S. Nuamtanong, T. Kusolsuk, M. Chairoj, P. T. Yenchitsomanas, and U. Chaisri. 2013. "Non-encapsulated *Trichinella* spp., *T. papuae*, diminishes severity of DSS-induced colitis in mice." *Asian Pac J Allergy Immunol* 31 (2):106-14. doi: 10.12932/AP0238.31.2.2013.

[28] Elliott, D. E., T. Setiawan, A. Metwali, A. Blum, J. F. Urban, Jr., and J. V. Weinstock. 2004. "*Heligmosomoides polygyrus* inhibits established colitis in IL-10-deficient mice." *Eur J Immunol* 34 (10):2690-8. doi: 10.1002/eji.200324833.

[29] Elliott, D. E., A. Metwali, J. Leung, T. Setiawan, A. M. Blum, M. N. Ince, L. E. Bazzone, M. J. Stadecker, J. F. Urban, Jr., and J. V. Weinstock. 2008. "Colonization with *Heligmosomoides polygyrus* suppresses mucosal IL-17 production." *J Immunol* 181 (4):2414-9. doi: 10.4049/jimmunol.181.4.2414.

[30] Metwali, A., T. Setiawan, A. M. Blum, J. Urban, D. E. Elliott, L. Hang, and J. V. Weinstock. 2006. "Induction of CD8+ regulatory T cells in the intestine by *Heligmosomoides polygyrus* infection." *Am J*

Physiol Gastrointest Liver Physiol 291 (2):G253-9. doi: 10.1152/ajpgi.00409.2005.

[31] Blum, A. M., L. Hang, T. Setiawan, J. P. Urban, Jr., K. M. Stoyanoff, J. Leung, and J. V. Weinstock. 2012. "*Heligmosomoides polygyrus* bakeri induces tolerogenic dendritic cells that block colitis and prevent antigen-specific gut T cell responses." *J Immunol* 189 (5):2512-20. doi: 10.4049/jimmunol.1102892.

[32] Donskow-Lysoniewska, K., P. Majewski, K. Brodaczewska, K. Jozwicka, and M. Doligalska. 2012. "*Heligmosmoides polygyrus* fourth stages induce protection against DSS-induced colitis and change opioid expression in the intestine." *Parasite Immunol* 34 (11):536-46. doi: 10.1111/pim.12003.

[33] Moreels, T. G., R. J. Nieuwendijk, J. G. De Man, B. Y. De Winter, A. G. Herman, E. A. Van Marck, and P. A. Pelckmans. 2004. "Concurrent infection with *Schistosoma mansoni* attenuates inflammation induced changes in colonic morphology, cytokine levels, and smooth muscle contractility of trinitrobenzene sulphonic acid induced colitis in rats." *Gut* 53 (1):99-107. doi: 10.1136/gut.53.1.99.

[34] Smith, P., N. E. Mangan, C. M. Walsh, R. E. Fallon, A. N. McKenzie, N. van Rooijen, and P. G. Fallon. 2007. "Infection with a helminth parasite prevents experimental colitis via a macrophage-mediated mechanism." *J Immunol* 178 (7):4557 66. doi: 10.4049/jimmunol.178.7.4557.

[35] Bodammer, P., C. Maletzki, G. Waitz, and J. Emmrich. 2011. "Prophylactic application of bovine colostrum ameliorates murine colitis via induction of immunoregulatory cells." *J Nutr* 141 (6):1056-61. doi: 10.3945/jn.110.128702.

[36] Elliott, D. E., J. Li, A. Blum, A. Metwali, K. Qadir, J. F. Urban, Jr., and J. V. Weinstock. 2003. "Exposure to schistosome eggs protects mice from TNBS-induced colitis." *Am J Physiol Gastrointest Liver Physiol* 284 (3):G385-91. doi: 10.1152/ajpgi.00049.2002.

[37] Zhao, Y., S. Zhang, L. Jiang, J. Jiang, and H. Liu. 2009. "Preventive effects of Schistosoma japonicum ova on trinitrobenzenesulfonic

acid-induced colitis and bacterial translocation in mice." *J Gastroenterol Hepatol* 24 (11):1775-80. doi: 10.1111/j.1440-1746.2009.05986.x.

[38] Hunter, M. M., A. Wang, C. L. Hirota, and D. M. McKay. 2005. "Neutralizing anti-IL-10 antibody blocks the protective effect of tapeworm infection in a murine model of chemically induced colitis." *J Immunol* 174 (11):7368-75. doi: 10.4049/jimmunol.174.11.7368.

[39] Bodammer, P., G. Waitz, M. Loebermann, M. C. Holtfreter, C. Maletzki, M. R. Krueger, H. Nizze, J. Emmrich, and E. C. Reisinger. 2011. "*Schistosoma mansoni* infection but not egg antigen promotes recovery from colitis in outbred NMRI mice." *Dig Dis Sci* 56 (1):70-8. doi: 10.1007/s10620-010-1237-y.

[40] Leung, J., L. Hang, A. Blum, T. Setiawan, K. Stoyanoff, and J. Weinstock. 2012. "*Heligmosomoides polygyrus* abrogates antigen-specific gut injury in a murine model of inflammatory bowel disease." *Inflamm Bowel Dis* 18 (8):1447-55. doi: 10.1002/ibd.22858.

[41] Summers, R. W., D. E. Elliott, K. Qadir, J. F. Urban, Jr., R. Thompson, and J. V. Weinstock. 2003. "*Trichuris suis* seems to be safe and possibly effective in the treatment of inflammatory bowel disease." *Am J Gastroenterol* 98 (9):2034-41. doi: 10.1111/j.1572-0241.2003.07660.x.

[42] Summers, R. W., D. E. Elliott, J. F. Urban, Jr., R. Thompson, and J. V. Weinstock. 2005. "*Trichuris suis* therapy in Crohn's disease." *Gut* 54 (1):87-90. doi: 10.1136/gut.2004.041749.

[43] Summers, R. W., D. E. Elliott, J. F. Urban, Jr., R. A. Thompson, and J. V. Weinstock. 2005. "*Trichuris suis* therapy for active ulcerative colitis: a randomized controlled trial." *Gastroenterology* 128 (4):825-32. doi: 10.1053/j.gastro.2005.01.005.

[44] Croese, J., J. O'Neil, J. Masson, S. Cooke, W. Melrose, D. Pritchard, and R. Speare. 2006. "A proof of concept study establishing *Necator americanus* in Crohn's patients and reservoir donors." *Gut* 55 (1):136-7. doi: 10.1136/gut.2005.079129.

[45] Sandborn, W. J., D. E. Elliott, J. Weinstock, R. W. Summers, A. Landry-Wheeler, N. Silver, M. D. Harnett, and S. B. Hanauer. 2013.

"Randomised clinical trial: the safety and tolerability of *Trichuris suis ova* in patients with Crohn's disease." *Aliment Pharmacol Ther* 38 (3):255-63. doi: 10.1111/apt.12366.

[46] Sobotkova, K., W. Parker, J. Leva, J. Ruzkova, J. Lukes, and K. Jirku Pomajbikova. 2019. "Helminth Therapy - From the Parasite Perspective." *Trends Parasitol* 35 (7):501-515. doi: 10.1016/j.pt.2019.04.009.

[47] Kahl, J., N. Brattig, and E. Liebau. 2018. "The Untapped Pharmacopeic Potential of Helminths." *Trends Parasitol* 34 (10):828-842. doi: 10.1016/j.pt.2018.05.011.

[48] Hepworth, M. R., and S. Hartmann. 2012. "Worming our way closer to the clinic." *Int J Parasitol Drugs Drug Resist* 2:187-90. doi: 10.1016/j.ijpddr.2012.07.001.

[49] Togre, N., P. Bhoj, K. Goswami, A. Tarnekar, M. Patil, and M. Shende. 2018. "Human filarial proteins attenuate chronic colitis in an experimental mouse model." *Parasite Immunol* 40 (3). doi: 10.1111/pim.12511.

[50] Zakeri, A., E. P. Hansen, S. D. Andersen, A. R. Williams, and P. Nejsum. 2018. "Immunomodulation by Helminths: Intracellular Pathways and Extracellular Vesicles." *Front Immunol* 9:2349. doi: 10.3389/fimmu.2018.02349.

[51] Ruyssers, N. E., B. Y. De Winter, J. G. De Man, A. Loukas, M. S. Pearson, J. V. Weinstock, R. M. Van den Bussche, W. Martinet, P. A. Pelckmans, and T. G. Moreels. 2009. "Therapeutic potential of helminth soluble proteins in TNBS-induced colitis in mice." *Inflamm Bowel Dis* 15 (4):491-500. doi: 10.1002/ibd.20787.

[52] Motomura, Y., H. Wang, Y. Deng, R. T. El-Sharkawy, E. F. Verdu, and W. I. Khan. 2009. "Helminth antigen-based strategy to ameliorate inflammation in an experimental model of colitis." *Clin Exp Immunol* 155 (1):88-95. doi: 10.1111/j.1365-2249.2008.03805.x.

[53] Johnston, M. J., A. Wang, M. E. Catarino, L. Ball, V. C. Phan, J. A. MacDonald, and D. M. McKay. 2010. "Extracts of the rat tapeworm, *Hymenolepis diminuta*, suppress macrophage activation in vitro and

alleviate chemically induced colitis in mice." *Infect Immun* 78 (3):1364-75. doi: 10.1128/IAI.01349-08.

[54] Cancado, G. G., J. A. Fiuza, N. C. de Paiva, C. Lemos Lde, N. D. Ricci, P. H. Gazzinelli-Guimaraes, V. G. Martins, D. C. Bartholomeu, D. A. Negrao-Correa, C. M. Carneiro, and R. T. Fujiwara. 2011. "Hookworm products ameliorate dextran sodium sulfate-induced colitis in BALB/c mice." *Inflamm Bowel Dis* 17 (11):2275-86. doi: 10.1002/ibd.21629.

[55] Ferreira, I., D. Smyth, S. Gaze, A. Aziz, P. Giacomin, N. Ruyssers, D. Artis, T. Laha, S. Navarro, A. Loukas, and H. J. McSorley. 2013. "Hookworm excretory/secretory products induce interleukin-4 (IL-4)+ IL-10+ CD4+ T cell responses and suppress pathology in a mouse model of colitis." *Infect Immun* 81 (6):2104-11. doi: 10.1128/IAI.00563-12.

[56] Heylen, M., N. E. Ruyssers, J. G. De Man, J. P. Timmermans, P. A. Pelckmans, T. G. Moreels, and B. Y. De Winter. 2014. "Worm proteins of Schistosoma mansoni reduce the severity of experimental chronic colitis in mice by suppressing colonic proinflammatory immune responses." *PLoS One* 9 (10):e110002. doi: 10.1371/journal.pone.0110002.

[57] Harnett, W., and M. M. Harnett. 2009. "Immunomodulatory activity and therapeutic potential of the filarial nematode secreted product, ES-62." *Adv Exp Med Biol* 666:88-94. doi: 10.1007/978-1-4419-1601-3_7.

[58] Zaccone, P., O. T. Burton, S. E. Gibbs, N. Miller, F. M. Jones, G. Schramm, H. Haas, M. J. Doenhoff, D. W. Dunne, and A. Cooke. 2011. "The S. mansoni glycoprotein omega-1 induces Foxp3 expression in NOD mouse CD4(+) T cells." *Eur J Immunol* 41 (9):2709-18. doi: 10.1002/eji.201141429.

[59] Manoury, B., W. F. Gregory, R. M. Maizels, and C. Watts. 2001. "Bm-CPI-2, a cystatin homolog secreted by the filarial parasite *Brugia malayi*, inhibits class II MHC-restricted antigen processing." *Curr Biol* 11 (6):447-51. doi: 10.1016/s0960-9822(01)00118-x.

[60] Pfaff, A. W., H. Schulz-Key, P. T. Soboslay, D. W. Taylor, K. MacLennan, and W. H. Hoffmann. 2002. "*Litomosoides sigmodontis* cystatin acts as an immunomodulator during experimental filariasis." *Int J Parasitol* 32 (2):171-8.

[61] Schonemeyer, A., R. Lucius, B. Sonnenburg, N. Brattig, R. Sabat, K. Schilling, J. Bradley, and S. Hartmann. 2001. "Modulation of human T cell responses and macrophage functions by onchocystatin, a secreted protein of the filarial nematode *Onchocerca volvulus*." *J Immunol* 167 (6):3207-15. doi: 10.4049/jimmunol.167.6.3207.

[62] Hartmann, S., B. Kyewski, B. Sonnenburg, and R. Lucius. 1997. "A filarial cysteine protease inhibitor down-regulates T cell proliferation and enhances interleukin-10 production." *Eur J Immunol* 27 (9):2253-60. doi: 10.1002/eji.1830270920.

[63] Gabrijelcic, D., B. Svetic, D. Spaic, J. Skrk, M. Budihna, I. Dolenc, T. Popovic, V. Cotic, and V. Turk. 1992. "Cathepsins B, H and L in human breast carcinoma." *Eur J Clin Chem Clin Biochem* 30 (2): 69-74.

[64] Lenarcic, B., J. Kos, I. Dolenc, P. Lucovnik, I. Krizaj, and V. Turk. 1988. "Cathepsin D inactivates cysteine proteinase inhibitors, cystatins." *Biochem Biophys Res Commun* 154 (2):765-72. doi: 10.1016/0006-291x(88)90206-9.

[65] Trabandt, A., W. K. Aicher, R. E. Gay, V. P. Sukhatme, M. Nilson-Hamilton, R. T. Hamilton, J. R. McGhee, H. G. Fassbender, and S. Gay. 1990. "Expression of the collagenolytic and Ras-induced cysteine proteinase cathepsin L and proliferation-associated oncogenes in synovial cells of MRL/I mice and patients with rheumatoid arthritis." *Matrix* 10 (6):349-61.

[66] Brage, M., A. Lie, M. Ransjo, F. Kasprzykowski, R. Kasprzykowska, M. Abrahamson, A. Grubb, and U. H. Lerner, 2004. "Osteoclastogenesis is decreased by cysteine proteinase inhibitors." *Bone* 34 (3):412-24. doi: 10.1016/j.bone.2003.11.018.

[67] Ziegler, T., S. Rausch, S. Steinfelder, C. Klotz, M. R. Hepworth, A. A. Kuhl, P. C. Burda, R. Lucius, and S. Hartmann. 2015. "A novel regulatory macrophage induced by a helminth molecule instructs IL-

10 in CD4+ T cells and protects against mucosal inflammation." *J Immunol* 194 (4):1555-64. doi: 10.4049/jimmunol.1401217.

[68] Schnoeller, C., S. Rausch, S. Pillai, A. Avagyan, B. M. Wittig, C. Loddenkemper, A. Hamann, E. Hamelmann, R. Lucius, and S. Hartmann. 2008. "A helminth immunomodulator reduces allergic and inflammatory responses by induction of IL-10-producing macrophages." *J Immunol* 180 (6):4265-72. doi: 10.4049/jimmunol. 180.6.4265.

[69] Whelan, R. A., S. Rausch, F. Ebner, D. Gunzel, J. F. Richter, N. A. Hering, J. D. Schulzke, A. A. Kuhl, A. Keles, P. Janczyk, K. Nockler, L. H. Wieler, and S. Hartmann. 2014. "A transgenic probiotic secreting a parasite immunomodulator for site-directed treatment of gut inflammation." *Mol Ther* 22 (10):1730-40. doi: 10.1038/mt.2014.125.

[70] Wang, S., Y. Xie, X. Yang, X. Wang, K. Yan, Z. Zhong, X. Wang, Y. Xu, Y. Zhang, F. Liu, and J. Shen. 2016. "Therapeutic potential of recombinant cystatin from *Schistosoma japonicum* in TNBS-induced experimental colitis of mice." *Parasit Vectors* 9:6. doi: 10.1186/s13071-015-1288-1.

[71] Coronado, S., L. Barrios, J. Zakzuk, R. Regino, V. Ahumada, L. Franco, Y. Ocampo, and L. Caraballo. 2017. "A recombinant cystatin from *Ascaris lumbricoides* attenuates inflammation of DSS-induced colitis." *Parasite Immunol* 39 (4). doi: 10.1111/pim.12425.

[72] Jang, S. W., M. K. Cho, M. K. Park, S. A. Kang, B. K. Na, S. C. Ahn, D. H. Kim, and H. S. Yu. 2011. "Parasitic helminth cystatin inhibits DSS-induced intestinal inflammation via IL-10(+)F4/80(+) macrophage recruitment." *Korean J Parasitol* 49 (3):245-54. doi: 10.3347/kjp.2011.49.3.245.

[73] Xu, J., M. Liu, P. Yu, L. Wu, and Y. Lu. 2019. "Effect of recombinant *Trichinella spiralis* cysteine proteinase inhibitor on TNBS-induced experimental inflammatory bowel disease in mice." *Int Immunopharmacol* 66:28-40. doi: 10.1016/j.intimp.2018.10.043.

[74] Khatri, V., N. Amdare, A. Tarnekar, K. Goswami, and M. V. Reddy. 2015. "*Brugia malayi* cystatin therapeutically ameliorates dextran

sulfate sodium-induced colitis in mice." *J Dig Dis* 16 (10):585-94. doi: 10.1111/1751-2980.12290.

[75] Schierack, P., R. Lucius, B. Sonnenburg, K. Schilling, and S. Hartmann. 2003. "Parasite-specific immunomodulatory functions of filarial cystatin." *Infect Immun* 71 (5):2422-9. doi: 10.1128/iai.71.5.2422-2429.2003.

[76] O'Regan, N. L., S. Steinfelder, G. Venugopal, G. B. Rao, R. Lucius, A. Srikantam, and S. Hartmann. 2014. "Brugia malayi microfilariae induce a regulatory monocyte/macrophage phenotype that suppresses innate and adaptive immune responses." *PLoS Negl Trop Dis* 8 (10):e3206. doi: 10.1371/journal.pntd.0003206.

[77] Semnani, R. T., M. Law, J. Kubofcik, and T. B. Nutman. 2004. "Filaria-induced immune evasion: suppression by the infective stage of Brugia malayi at the earliest host-parasite interface." *J Immunol* 172 (10):6229-38. doi: 10.4049/jimmunol.172.10.6229.

[78] Du, L., H. Tang, Z. Ma, J. Xu, W. Gao, J. Chen, W. Gan, Z. Zhang, X. Yu, X. Zhou, and X. Hu. 2011. "The protective effect of the recombinant 53-kDa protein of *Trichinella spiralis* on experimental colitis in mice." *Dig Dis Sci* 56 (10):2810-7. doi: 10.1007/s10620-011-1689-8.

[79] Cho, M. K., C. H. Lee, and H. S. Yu. 2011. "Amelioration of intestinal colitis by macrophage migration inhibitory factor isolated from intestinal parasites through toll-like receptor 2." *Parasite Immunol* 33 (5):265-75. doi: 10.1111/j.1365-3024.2010.01276.x.

[80] Khatri, V., N. Amdare, R. S. Yadav, A. Tarnekar, K. Goswami, and M. V. Reddy. 2015. "*Brugia malayi* abundant larval transcript 2 protein treatment attenuates experimentally-induced colitis in mice." *Indian J Exp Biol* 53 (11):732-9.

[81] Kron, M. A., A. Metwali, S. Vodanovic-Jankovic, and D. Elliott. 2013. "Nematode asparaginyl-tRNA synthetase resolves intestinal inflammation in mice with T-cell transfer colitis." *Clin Vaccine Immunol* 20 (2):276-81. doi: 10.1128/CVI.00594-12.

[82] Kim, J. Y., M. K. Cho, S. H. Choi, K. H. Lee, S. C. Ahn, D. H. Kim, and H. S. Yu. 2010. "Inhibition of dextran sulfate sodium (DSS)-

induced intestinal inflammation via enhanced IL-10 and TGF-beta production by galectin-9 homologues isolated from intestinal parasites." *Mol Biochem Parasitol* 174 (1):53-61. doi: 10.1016/j.molbiopara.2010.06.014.

[83] Du, L., H. Wei, L. Li, H. Shan, Y. Yu, Y. Wang, and G. Zhang. 2014. "Regulation of recombinant *Trichinella spiralis* 53-kDa protein (rTsP53) on alternatively activated macrophages via STAT6 but not IL-4Ralpha in vitro." *Cell Immunol* 288 (1-2):1-7. doi: 10.1016/j.cellimm.2014.01.010.

[84] Mendlovic, F., M. Cruz-Rivera, J. A. Diaz-Gandarilla, M. A. Flores-Torres, G. Avila, M. Perfiliev, A. M. Salazar, L. Arriaga-Pizano, P. Ostrosky-Wegman, and A. Flisser. 2017. "Orally administered *Taenia solium* Calreticulin prevents experimental intestinal inflammation and is associated with a type 2 immune response." *PLoS One* 12 (10):e0186510. doi: 10.1371/journal.pone.0186510.

[85] Wang, L., H. Xie, L. Xu, Q. Liao, S. Wan, Z. Yu, D. Lin, B. Zhang, Z. Lv, Z. Wu, and X. Sun. 2017. "rSj16 Protects against DSS-Induced Colitis by Inhibiting the PPAR-alpha Signaling Pathway." *Theranostics* 7 (14):3446-3460. doi: 10.7150/thno.20359.

[86] Driss, V., M. El Nady, M. Delbeke, C. Rousseaux, C. Dubuquoy, A. Sarazin, S. Gatault, A. Dendooven, G. Riveau, J. F. Colombel, P. Desreumaux, L. Dubuquoy, and M. Capron. 2016. "The schistosome glutathione S-transferase P28GST, a unique helminth protein, prevents intestinal inflammation in experimental colitis through a Th2-type response with mucosal eosinophils." *Mucosal Immunol* 9 (2):322-35. doi: 10.1038/mi.2015.62.

[87] Thi, T. H. H., P. A. Priemel, Y. Karrout, V. Driss, M. Delbeke, A. Dendooven, M. P. Flament, M. Capron, and J. Siepmann. 2017. "Preparation and investigation of P28GST-loaded PLGA microparticles for immunomodulation of experimental colitis." *Int J Pharm* 533 (1):26-33. doi: 10.1016/j.ijpharm.2017.09.037.

[88] Sarazin, A., A. Dendooven, M. Delbeke, S. Gatault, A. Pagny, A. Standaert, C. Rousseaux, P. Desreumaux, L. Dubuquoy, and M. Capron. 2018. "Treatment with P28GST, a schistosome-derived

enzyme, after acute colitis induction in mice: Decrease of intestinal inflammation associated with a down regulation of Th1/Th17 responses." *PLoS One* 13 (12):e0209681. doi: 10.1371/journal.pone. 0209681.

[89] McKay, D. M. 2009. "The therapeutic helminth?" *Trends Parasitol* 25 (3):109-14. doi: 10.1016/j.pt.2008.11.008.

[90] Hubner, M. P., Y. Shi, M. N. Torrero, E. Mueller, D. Larson, K. Soloviova, F. Gondorf, A. Hoerauf, K. E. Killoran, J. T. Stocker, S. J. Davies, K. V. Tarbell, and E. Mitre. 2012. "Helminth protection against autoimmune diabetes in nonobese diabetic mice is independent of a type 2 immune shift and requires TGF-beta." *J Immunol* 188 (2):559-68. doi: 10.4049/jimmunol.1100335.

[91] Setiawan, T., A. Metwali, A. M. Blum, M. N. Ince, J. F. Urban, Jr., D. E. Elliott, and J. V. Weinstock. 2007. "Heligmosomoides polygyrus promotes regulatory T-cell cytokine production in the murine normal distal intestine." *Infect Immun* 75 (9):4655-63. doi: 10.1128/IAI.00358-07.

[92] Eftychi, C., R. Schwarzer, K. Vlantis, L. Wachsmuth, M. Basic, P. Wagle, M. F. Neurath, C. Becker, A. Bleich, and M. Pasparakis. 2019. "Temporally Distinct Functions of the Cytokines IL-12 and IL-23 Drive Chronic Colon Inflammation in Response to Intestinal Barrier Impairment." *Immunity*. doi: 10.1016/j.immuni.2019.06.008.

[93] Cruickshank, J. M. 1992. "Clinical importance of coronary perfusion pressure in the hypertensive patient with left ventricular hypertrophy." *Cardiology* 81 (4-5):283-90. doi: 10.1159/000175818.

[94] Danilowicz-Luebert, E., S. Steinfelder, A. A. Kuhl, G. Drozdenko, R. Lucius, M. Worm, E. Hamelmann, and S. Hartmann. 2013. "A nematode immunomodulator suppresses grass pollen-specific allergic responses by controlling excessive Th2 inflammation." *Int J Parasitol* 43 (3-4):201-10. doi: 10.1016/j.ijpara.2012.10.014.

[95] Matisz, C. E., B. Faz-Lopez, E. Thomson, A. Al Rajabi, F. Lopes, L. I. Terrazas, A. Wang, K. A. Sharkey, and D. M. McKay. 2017. "Suppression of colitis by adoptive transfer of helminth antigen-

treated dendritic cells requires interleukin-4 receptor-alpha signaling." *Sci Rep* 7:40631. doi: 10.1038/srep40631.

[96] Reyes, J. L., A. Wang, M. R. Fernando, R. Graepel, G. Leung, N. van Rooijen, M. Sigvardsson, and D. M. McKay. 2015. "Splenic B cells from *Hymenolepis diminuta*-infected mice ameliorate colitis independent of T cells and via cooperation with macrophages." *J Immunol* 194 (1):364-78. doi: 10.4049/jimmunol.1400738.

[97] Kang, S. A., M. K. Park, S. K. Park, J. H. Choi, D. I. Lee, S. M. Song, and H. S. Yu. 2019. "Adoptive transfer of *Trichinella spiralis*-activated macrophages can ameliorate both Th1- and Th2-activated inflammation in murine models." *Sci Rep* 9 (1):6547. doi: 10.1038/s41598-019-43057-1.

[98] Vermeire, J. J., Y. Cho, E. Lolis, R. Bucala, and M. Cappello. 2008. "Orthologs of macrophage migration inhibitory factor from parasitic nematodes." *Trends Parasitol* 24 (8):355-63. doi: 10.1016/j.pt.2008.04.007.

[99] Cho, M. K., M. K. Park, S. A. Kang, S. K. Park, J. H. Lyu, D. H. Kim, H. K. Park, and H. S. Yu. 2015. "TLR2-dependent amelioration of allergic airway inflammation by parasitic nematode type II MIF in mice." *Parasite Immunol* 37 (4):180-91. doi: 10.1111/pim.12172.

[100] Taghipour, N., H. A. Aghdaei, A. Haghighi, N. Mossafa, S. J. Tabaei, and M. Rostami-Nejad. 2014. "Potential treatment of inflammatory bowel disease: a review of helminths therapy." *Gastroenterol Hepatol Bed Bench* 7 (1):9-16.

[101] Marchioni Beery, R., and S. Kane. 2014. "Current approaches to the management of new-onset ulcerative colitis." *Clin Exp Gastroenterol* 7:111-32. doi: 10.2147/CEG.S35942.

[102] Buning, C., and H. Lochs. 2006. "Conventional therapy for Crohn's disease." *World J Gastroenterol* 12 (30):4794-806.

[103] Thai, A., and T. Prindiville. 2010. "Hepatosplenic T-cell lymphoma and inflammatory bowel disease." *J Crohns Colitis* 4 (5):511-22. doi: 10.1016/j.crohns.2010.05.006.

[104] Monaco, C., J. Nanchahal, P. Taylor, and M. Feldmann. 2015. "Anti-TNF therapy: past, present and future." *Int Immunol* 27 (1):55-62. doi: 10.1093/intimm/dxu102.

BIOGRAPHICAL SKETCHES

Kalyan Goswami

Affiliation: Professor, Department of Biochemistry

Education: MD (Biochemistry)

Research and Professional Experience:

Area of research interest involves oxidative and glycative stress, apoptotic impact and immune modulation for drug development, metabolic stress and application of bio-statistics in quality control of clinical chemistry and educational research on non-conventional and integrated teaching. Earlier work on detection of auto-antibody against mannose binding lectin (MBL) as Scientist in Council of Scientific and Industrial Research (CSIR) led to development of a diagnostic kit for rheumatoid arthritis. Certain herbal polyphenolics and their synthetic analogs has been validated that might be used to treat filariasis and also further exploration of novel approach exploiting targeted apoptosis has been carried out. Our work successfully demonstrated silver nano-particle as the unique therapeutic lead based on apoptotic rationale. Bioinformatics based detection and validation of target with its potential role in pathogenesis has been successfully incorporated in the filarial drug research. I have worked as principal investigator in 'Study of interaction between platelet and human lymphatic filarial parasite with focus on eicosanoid metabolism and its pathophysiological implication' under SERB scheme of Department of Science & Technology, Govt. of India. I am also principal co-investigator in "Elusive role of HDL-C in metabolic syndrome and impending CVD" under SERB scheme of Department of Science & Technology, Govt. of India. Earlier I had completed projects as co-investigator in National Repository Project for filarial parasites and reagents under Department of Biotechnology, Govt. of India as well as in "Evaluation of immunomodulatory effect and therapeutic potential of Filarial proteins in experimental ulcerative colitis" under Department of Science & Technology, Govt. of India. I have published more than 70 articles with total citations of around 1100 and also one international and one national patent to my credit.

Professional Appointments:

2001 – 2004	Senior Resident Department of Biochemistry, JIPMER, Puducherry. & JB Tropical Disease Research Center, Mahatma Gandhi Institute of Medical Sciences, Sevagram, India.
2004 - 2005	Scientist, Institute of Genomics & Integrative Biology, Delhi under Council for Scientific & Industrial Research, Govt. Of India.
2005-2007	Assistant Professor, Department of Biochemistry & JB Tropical Disease Research Center, Mahatma Gandhi Institute of Medical Sciences, Sevagram, India.
2007 - 2011	Associate Professor, Department of Biochemistry & JB Tropical Disease Research Center, Mahatma Gandhi Institute of Medical Sciences, Sevagram, India.
2011-2018	Professor, Department of Biochemistry & JB Tropical Disease Research Center, Mahatma Gandhi Institute of Medical Sciences, Sevagram, India.
2018-2019	Additional Professor, Department of Biochemistry, AIIMS, Raipur, India.
2019 July onwards	Professor & Head, Department of Biochemistry, AIIMS, Kalyani, India.

Publications from the Last 3 Years:

1. Amdare NP, Khatri VK, Yadav RS, Tarnekar A, Goswami K, Reddy MV. Therapeutic potential of immunomodulatory proteins *Wuchereria bancrofti* L2 and *Brugia malayi* abundant larval transcript 2 against STZ-induced type 1 diabetes in mice." *J Helminthol.* 2016; 26:1-10.
2. Mandvikar A., Hande S., Yeole P., Goswami K., Reddy M. V. R. Therapeutic potential of novel heterocyclic thiazolidine compounds against human lymphatic filarial parasite: an *in vitro* study.' *IJPSR.* (2016); 7(4): 1480-1492.
3. Hande S, Goswami K, Bhoj P, Mandvikar A, Reddy MVR. Oxidative Stress Induced Apoptosis by Thiazolidine Compounds: A Unique Antifilarial Approach. *SMU Medical Journal*, (2016); 3(1):685-696.
4. Yadav R S P, Khatri V, Amdare N, Goswami K, Shivkumar V. B., Gangane N, Reddy M V R. Immuno-Modulatory Effect and Therapeutic Potential of *Brugia malayi* Cystatin in Experimentally Induced Arthritis. *Ind. J. Clin. Biochem.* (2016); 31(2): 203-8.
5. Kamble P., Goswami K.. Microalbuminuria: A mere Marker or An Ominous Sign?" *Journal of the Association of Physicians of India*. (2016); 64: 61-65.
6. . Bahekar S P, Hande S V., Agrawal N R., Chandak H S., Bhoj P S., Goswami K, Reddy M. V. R.. Sulfonamide Chalcones: Synthesis and in vitro exploration for therapeutic potential against *Brugia Malayi*. *European Journal of Medicinal Chemistry*. (2016)124; 262-269.
7. Hande S, Goswami K, Togre N, Mandvikar A, Reddy M. V. R. Antifilarial actions of green tea extract and a synthetic heterocyclic thiazolidine derivative, Im8 compound in experimental mouse model. *Indian Journal of Experimental Biology* (2016); 54: 753-757.
8. Reddy S. M., Reddy P. M., Amdare N, Khatri V, Tarnekar A, Goswami K, Reddy MVR. Filarial Abundant Larval Transcript

Protein ALT-2: An Immunomodulatory Therapeutic Agent for Type 1 Diabetes. *Ind J Clin Biochem* (2017) 32 (1): 45-52.
9. Togre N S., Bhoj P S., Khatri V K., Tarnekar A, Goswami K, Shende M R., Reddy MVR. SXP–RAL Family Filarial Protein, rWbL2, prevents development of DSS-induced acute ulcerative colitis. *Ind. J. Clin. Biochem.* (2017) 1-8.
10. Yadav R S P, Khatri V, Amdare N, Goswami K, Shivkumar VB, Gangane N, Reddy M V R. Evaluation of preventive effect of Brugia malayi recombinant cystatin on mBSA-induced experimental arthritis. *Indian Journal of Experimental Biology.* (2017) 55: 655-660;
11. Bhoj P, Togre N, Bahekar S, Goswami K, Chandak H, Patil M. Immunomodulatory activity of sulfonamide chalcone compounds in mice infected with filarial parasite, Brugia malayi *Ind. J. Clin. Biochem.* (2018) 1-5,
12. Bhoj PS, Ingle RG, Goswami K, Jena L, Wadher S. Apoptotic impact on *Brugia malayi* by sulphonamido-quinoxaline: search for a novel therapeutic rationale. *Parasitol Res.* (2018); 17(5):1559-1572.
13. Togre N, Bhoj P, Goswami K, A Tarnekar, Patil M, Shende M. Human filarial proteins attenuate chronic colitis in an experimental mouse model. *Parasite Immunology.* (2018); 40:e12511.
14. Togre N, Bhoj P, Amdare N, Goswami K, Tarnekar A, Shende M. Immunomodulatory potential of recombinant filarial protein, rWbL2 and its therapeutic implication in experimental ulcerative colitis in mouse. *Immunopharmacology and Immunotoxicology.* (2018); 1-8.
15. Goswami K, Gandhe M. Evolution of metabolic syndrome and its biomarkers. *Diabetes & Metabolic Syndrome: Clinical Research & Reviews.* (2018); S1871-4021(18): 30232-7.

16. Togre N, Khatri V, Nakhale M, Bhoj P, Goswami K, Tarnekar A, Patil M, Kumar S. Exploration of immune modulation by combination of filarial proteins against DSS induced colitis in mouse mode. *Romanian Archives of Microbiology and Immunology*. (2018); 77 (2): 65-80.
17. Prasad B V S, Khatri V Yadav R P S, Chandra M S, Vijayalakshmi D, Goswami K. Immunodiagnostic potential of Wuchereria bancrofti L1 antigen–based filarial immunoglobulin G4 detection assay. *Transactions of The Royal Society of Tropical Medicine and Hygiene*. (2019); 113 (1): 36-43.
18. Manupati K., Debnath B., Goswami K., Rhoya P., Chandak H., Bahekar S., Das A. Glutathione-S-transferase omega 1 inhibition activates JNK-mediated apoptotic response in breast cancer stem cells. FEBS Journal. *The FEBS Journal*. (2019); 286: 2167–2192.
19. Palaniswamy R, Goswami K, Nandakumar DN, Srinivas D, Chandrajit P. TNF-α mediated MEK-ERK signaling in invasion with putative network involving NF-κB and STAT-6: a new perspective in glioma. *Cell Biology International*.
20. Bhoj P, Togre N, K Goswami, V Madhariya. Polyphenols-Induced Apoptosis by *Murraya koenigii* against lymphatic filarial parasite and its therapeutic implication. *Journal of Herbs, Spices & Medicinal Plants*. (2019). DOI:10.1080/10496475.2019.1633454.
21. Waghmare P, Lende T, Goswami K, Gupta A, Gupta A, Gangane N, Kumar S. Immunological host responses as surveillance and prognostic markers in tubercular infections. *Int J Mycobacteriol*. 2019; 8:190-5.
22. Palaniswamy R, Goswami K, Nandakumar DN, Srinivas D, Chandrajit P. Survival of glioblastoma cells in response to endogenous and exogenous oxidative challenges: Possible implication of NMDA receptor mediated regulation of redox homeostasis. *Cell Biology International*. (in press).

Namdev S. Togre

Affiliation: Department of Hepatitis, National Institute of Virology, Pune, MH, India

Education: PhD Biochemistry

Research and Professional Experience:

Author did his Ph.D. in Biochemistry, especially in the exploration of therapeutic efficacy of filarial derived recombinant proteins against DSS acute and chronic colitis in mouse models. He has several research papers to his credit. His present interest centers on the generation of neutralizing monoclonal antibodies against Hepatitis E virus. He is presently working as a Research Associate in the Hepatitis Department, National Institute of Virology. Pune, MH, India.

Professional Appointments: Research Associate

Honors:

1. Babasaheb Ambedkar National Research Fellowship for Ph.D. research by Dr. Babasaheb Ambedkar Research & Training Institute (BARTI), Pune, Maharashtra, India for the year April 2015- Feb 2018.
2. Best Oral Paper Award at the 10th National conference of Indian Academy of Tropical Parasitology (TROPACON-2016) held at JIPMER, Pondicherry, during 2-6 Nov 2016.

Publications from the Last 3 Years:

1. Togre N, Bhoj P, Goswami K, Tarnekar A, Patil M, Shende M. Human filarial proteins attenuate chronic colitis in an experimental mouse model. *Parasite immunology*. 2018 March; 40 (3):e12511.

2. Togre N, Bhoj P, Amdare N, Goswami K, Tarnekar A, Shende M. Immunomodulatory potential of recombinant filarial protein, rWbL2, and its therapeutic implication in experimental ulcerative colitis in mouse. *Immunopharmacology and immunotoxicology*. 2018 Feb; 8:1-8.
3. Togre NS, Bhoj PS, Khatri VK, Tarnekar A, Goswami K, Shende MR, Reddy MV. SXP–RAL Family Filarial Protein, rWbL2, Prevents Development of DSS-Induced Acute Ulcerative Colitis. *Indian Journal of Clinical Biochemistry*. 2018 March; 33:282-289.
4. Togre N, Khatri V, Nakhale M, Bhoj P, Goswami K, Tarnekar A, Patil M, Kumar S. Exploration of immune modulation by combination of filarial proteins against DSS induced colitis in mouse model. *Romanian Archives of Microbiology and Immunology*. 2018 Aug; 77 (2): 65-80.
5. Khatri V, Amdare N, Chauhan N, Togre N, Reddy MV, Hoti SL, Kalyanasundaram R. Epidemiological screening and xenomonitoring for human lymphatic filariasis infection in select districts in the states of Maharashtra and Karnataka, India. *Parasitology research*. 2019 Mar 14;118 (3):1045-50.
6. Bhoj P, Togre N, Bahekar S, Goswami K, Chandak H, Patil M. Immunomodulatory Activity of Sulfonamide Chalcone Compounds in Mice Infected with Filarial Parasite, *Brugia malayi*. *Indian Journal of Clinical Biochemistry*. 2019 Apr 1,34 (2):225 9.
7. Hande S, Goswami K, Togre N, Mandvikar A, Reddy MVR. Antifilarial actions of green tea extract and a synthetic heterocyclic thiazolidine derivative, Im8 compound in experimental mouse model. *Indian Journal of Experimental Biology* 54, Nov 2016, 753 757
8. Bhoj P, Togre N, Goswami K, Madhariya V. Polyphenols-Induced Apoptosis by *Murraya Koenigii* against Lymphatic Filarial Parasite and Its Therapeutic Implication. *Journal of Herbs, Spices & Medicinal Plants*. 2019 Jul 14:1-4.

9. Bhoj P*, Daberao S, Togre N, Goswami K. Antifilarial and apoptotic effect of *Cardiospermum helicacabum* leaf extract on filarial *Brugia malayi* parasite. *Romanian Archives of Microbiology and Immunology*. 2018 Oct; 77 (4):294-300, *2018*.

Nitin P Amdare

Affiliation: Department of Microbiology and Immunology, Albert Einstein College of Medicine, Bronx, NY-10461

Education: MSc, PhD

Research and Professional Experience:

My primary career goal is to understand in detail the exact cellular and molecular mechanism involve in type 1 diabetes immunology and to develop safe therapeutic intervention in the treatment of type 1 diabetes. My academic training and research have provided an excellent background in multiple biological disciplines including Molecular biology, Biochemistry, Biotechnology and Immunology. My interest in life science research began when I had joined Dr. MVR Reddy's lab for short term dissertation during my M.Sc. studies, where, I had an opportunity to conduct research on diagnostic evaluation of filariasis using cocktail of filarial derived recombinant proteins. This experience introduced me to basic research as a career path and prompted me to join PhD programme in Dr. Reddy's lab at Mahatma Gandhi Institute of Medical Sciences. Initially, I started as a Research Fellow in Dr. Reddy's lab and my research was focused on the identification and development of the potential of filarial derived recombinant proteins and multivalent DNA, aimed at the development of filarial vaccines, drugs, and diagnostics.

More importantly, working on filarial research, during this period, I discovered the love working in the field of type 1 diabetes and learned that using filarial derived native or recombinant proteins to treat type 1 diabetes is an exceptionally novel and promising approach. This motivate me to continue working as a PhD graduate on the type 1 diabetes under the supervision of Dr. M. V. R. Reddy. During my PhD graduation tenure, I have published 02 first author research articles, 11 as a co-author and 02 are in communication and presented research work in many national and international scientific conferences. Fulfilment from doing excellent research in the field of type 1 diabetes inspired me to continue advance training as a scientist and pursue my postdoctoral research training in Dr. DiLorenzo lab at Albert Einstein College of medicine. Here, for my postdoctoral training, I continue to build my previous training in the therapeutics in type 1 diabetes translating into the humanized preclinical mouse model of type 1 diabetes will allow me to understand exact molecular and cellular mechanism and could lead us to discover safe therapeutic intervention for the T1D. My mentor and a sponsor Dr. Teresa DiLorenzo is an internationally well recognized and accomplished scientist in the fields of immunology and type 1 diabetes and has extensive record for training doctoral and postdoctoral fellows. Dr. DiLorenzo has been a leader in studies of NOD model of T1D and relevant to the proposed studies, has been involved in the characterization of humanized HLA transgenic NOD mice. My decision to work with laboratory of Dr. DiLorenzo prompted me to focus on the development of NOD mice transgenic for human insulin, a major autoantigen and expressing human MHC molecules in the system in order to identify the peptides derived from this autoantigen that are recognized by the islet-infiltrating CD8 T cells. In addition to this, currently, I am also working to develop humanized preclinical mouse model of T1D incorporating human beta cell-specific T cells (including hIns-specific ones), either engineered by lentiviral transduction or obtained from patients. Along with these projects, I am also working on the development of a methods to solve the crystal structure of T1D-associated class I MHC molecules.

Activity and Occupation	Start date (MM/YY)	Start date (M/YY)	Institute/Company	Supervisor/ Employer
MSc Intern	01/2009	03/2009	MGIMS, Sevagram, India	Dr. M. V. R. Reddy
Junior Research Fellow (DBT project)	10/2010	06/2014	MGIMS, Sevagram, India	Dr. M. V. R. Reddy
Senior Research Fellow (DBT project)	10/2014	03/2016	MGIMS, Sevagram, India	Dr. M. V. R. Reddy
PhD Scholar	10/2010	04/2017	MGIMS, Sevagram, India	Dr. M. V. R. Reddy
Research trainee	11/2016	04/2017	Albert Einstein College of Medicine, Bronx, NY	Dr. Teresa DiLorenzo
Postdoctoral Research Fellow	04/2017	Present	Albert Einstein College of Medicine, Bronx, NY	Dr. Teresa DiLorenzo

Professional Appointments:

Honors:

- ICMR International Travel Fellowship Govt. of India (for FOCIS 2014 Chicago, Illinois)
- Indian Immunology Society (IIS) bursary award

Publications from the Last 3 Years:

1. Khatri V, Amdare N, Chauhan N, Togre N, Reddy MV, Hoti SL, Kalyanasundaram R. Epidemiological screening and xenomonitoring for human lymphatic filariasis infection in select districts in the states of Maharashtra and Karnataka, India. *Parasitol Res.* 2019; 118(3):1045-1050.

2. Paul R, Ilamaran M, Khatri V, Amdare N, Reddy MVR, Kaliraj P. Immunological evaluation of fusion protein of *Brugia malayi* abundant larval protein transcript-2 (BmALT-2) and Tuftsin in experimental mice model. *Parasite Epidemiol Control.* 2019; 4:e00092. doi: 10.1016/j.parepi.2019.e00092.
3. Namdev Togre, Priyanka Bhoj, Nitin Amdare, Kalyan Goswami, Aaditya Tarnekar, Moreshwar Shende. Immunomodulatory potential of recombinant filarial protein, rWbL2, and its therapeutic implication in experimental ulcerative colitis in mouse. *Immunopharmacol Immunotoxicol.* 2018; 7:1-8. doi: 10.1080/08923973.2018.1431925.
4. Nitin Amdare, Vishal Khatri, Ravi Shankar Prasad Yadav, Aaditya Tarnekar, Kalyan Goswami, MVR Reddy. Therapeutic potential of immunomodulatory proteins *Wuchereria bancrofti* L2 and *Brugia malayi* abundant larval transcript 2 against STZ-induced type 1 diabetes in mice. *J Helminthol.* 2017;91(5):539-548.
5. Immanuel Christiana, Ramanathan Aparnaa, Balasubramaniyan Malathi, Khatri Vishal, Amdare Nitin, DN Rao, MVR Reddy & Kaliraj Perumal. Immunoprophylaxis of Multi-Antigen peptide (MAP) vaccine for Human lymphatic filariasis. *Immunologic Research.* 2017; 65(3):729-738. doi: 10.1007/s12026-017-8911-5.
6. Ravi Shankar Yadav, Vishal Khatri, Nitin Amdare, Kalyan Goswami, VB Shivkumar, Nitin Gangane, Maryada Venkata Rami Reddy. Evaluation of preventive effect of *Brugia malayi* recombinant cystatin on antigen-induced experimental arthritis. *Ind J exp Biochem.* 2016; 55:(655-660).
7. Sridhar M. Reddy, Pooja M. Reddy, Nitin Amdare, Vishal Khatri, Aaditya Tarnekar, Kalyan Goswami, Maryada Venkat Rami Reddy. Filarial Abundant Larval Transcript Protein ALT-2: An Immunomodulatory Therapeutic Agent for Type 1 Diabetes. *Indian J Clin Biochem.* 2017; 32(1):45-52.
8. Dhananjay Andure, Kiran Pote, Vishal Khatri, Nitin Amdare, Ramchandra Padalkar, Maryada Venkata Rami Reddy. "Immunization with *Wuchereria bancrofti* glutathione-s-

transferase elicits a mixed th1/th2 type of protective immune response against filarial infection in mastomys. *Ind J Clin Biochem. 2016;* 1-8.

Priyanka S Bhoj

Affiliation: Mahatma Gandhi Institute of Medical Sciences, Sevagram, MH, India

Education: PhD in Biochemistry

Research and Professional Experience:

Dr. Priyanka S. Bhoj did his Ph.D. in Biochemistry from Mahatma Gandhi Institute of Medical Sciences, Sevagram MH, India. Her research mainly focused on investigation of mechanism of apoptosis for designing therapeutic modality against *Brugia malayi*. She has published several research articles in journals of national and international repute.

Professional Appointments: PhD Fellow

Honors:

PS Murthy Best Oral paper award for the paper entitled 'Targeting folate metabolism: A promising therapeutic rationale against *Brugia malayi* infection' at 42nd ACBICON-2015 held at PGIMER, during 25-28 November, 2015.

Publications from the Last 3 Years:

1. Bhoj P, Ingle R, Goswami K, Wadher S. Apoptotic impact on *Brugia malayi* by sulphonamido-quinoxaline: search for a novel

therapeutic rationale. *Parasitology Research*. 2018; 117 (5): 1559-1572

2. Bhoj P, Togre N, Bahekar S, Goswami K, Chandak H, Patil M. Immunomodulatory activity of sulfonamide chalcone compounds in mice infected with filarial parasite, *Brugia malayi*. *Indian Journal of Clinical Biochemistry*. 2017: 1-5.

3. Bhoj P*, Daberao S, Togre N, Goswami K. Antifilarial and apoptotic effect of *Cardiospermum helicacabum* leaf extract on filarial *Brugia malayi* parasite. *Romanian Archives of Microbiology and Immunology*. 2018 Oct; 77 (4):294-300, *2018*. (*Corresponding author)

4. Bhoj P, Togre N, Goswami K, Madhariya V. Polyphenols-induced apoptosis by *Murraya koenigii* against lymphatic filarial parasite and its therapeutic implication. *Journal of Herbs, Spices and Medicinal Plants*. 2019 Jul 14:1-4.

5. Manupati K, Debnath S, Goswami K, Bhoj PS, Chandak HS, Bahekar SP, Das A. Glutathione S-transferase omega 1 inhibition activates JNK-mediated apoptotic response in breast cancer stem cells. *The FEBS journal*. 2019 Jun; 286 (11):2167-92.

6. Togre N, Bhoj P, Goswami K, Tarnekar A, Patil M, Shende M. Human filarial proteins attenuate chronic colitis in an experimental mouse model. *Parasite Immunology*. 2018; 40 (3): e12511.

7. Togre N, Bhoj P, Khatri V, Tarnekar A, Goswami K, Shende M. SXP-RAL family filarial protein, rWbL2, prevents development of DSS- induced acute ulcerative colitis. *Indian Journal of Clinical Biochemistry*. 2017; 33 (3): 282-9.

8. Togre N, Bhoj P, Amdare N, Goswami K, Tarnekar A, Shende M. Immunomodulatory potential of recombinant filarial protein, rWbL2 and its therapeutic implication in experimental ulcerative colitis in mouse. *Immunopharmacology and immunotoxicology. 2018 Feb; 8:1-8.*

9. Togre N, Khatri V, Nakhale M, Bhoj P, Goswami K, Tarnekar A, Shende M. Exploration of immune modulation by combination of filarial proteins against DSS induced acute colitis in mouse model.

Romanian Archives of Microbiology and Immunology. 2018 Aug; 77 (2): 65-80.
10. Bahekar S, Hande S, Agrawal N, Chandak H, Bhoj P, Goswami K, Reddy M. Sulfonamide chalcones: Synthesis and in vitro exploration for therapeutic potential against *Brugia malayi*. *European Journal of Medicinal Chemistry*. 2016; 124: 262-9.
11. Hande S, Goswami K, Sharma R, Bhoj P, Jena L, Reddy MV. Targeting folate metabolism for therapeutic option: A bioinformatics approach. *Indian Journal of Experimental Biology* 2015; 53: 762-766.
12. Goswami K, Hande S, Bhoj P, Jena L, Reddy MVR. Exploiting nanoparticle for targeted apoptosis as therapeutic modality against filarial parasite: A plausible premise. *OA Medical Hypothesis* 2014; 2 (2): 13.
13. Mahajan RS, Goswami K, Hande S, Bhoj P. Evolution of anti-filarial therapeutics: An overview. *Journal of Microbiology and Antimicrobial Agents*. 2015; 1(1).

Vishal Khatri

Affiliation: Postdoctoral Research Associate

Education: PhD Medical Biochemistry

Research and Professional Experience:

My research experience has been in development of helminth derived biotherapeutics for immune-mediated disorders, filarial vaccine and drug development. Part of this research has led to the identification of filarial-derived recombinant cystatin as a potential therapeutic molecule for the treatment of colitis, type 1 diabetes and rheumatoid arthritis. We have conducted research to uncover the underlying mechanism of action behind this therapeutic effect of cystatin and currently working towards identifying an active peptide moiety exhibiting therapeutic potential against colitis.

Furthermore, our research has led to the development of tetravalent fusion protein vaccine formulation *BmHAXT* for lymphatic filariasis, a disabling disease that affects over 140 million people in 72 different countries. The vaccine gave exciting protection of about 70% in rhesus macaques. The tetravalent lymphatic filariasis vaccine is currently under cGMP production for Phase I human clinical trials. I have published about 20 research articles with total citations of around 67 to my credit.

Professional Appointments:

2010 - 2014	Junior Research Fellow, Department of Biochemistry & JB Tropical Disease Research Center, Mahatma Gandhi Institute of Medical Sciences, Sevagram, India.
2014 - 2016	Senior Research Fellow, Department of Biochemistry & JB Tropical Disease Research Center, Mahatma Gandhi Institute of Medical Sciences, Sevagram, India.
2016 - 2017	Predoctoral Research Associate, University of Illinois College of Medicine, Rockford, IL.
2017 -	Postdoctoral Research Associate, University of Illinois College of Medicine, Rockford, IL.

Honors:

2007-2008	Deepa Biswas Memorial Best Student Award, Dr. Ambedkar College, India
2011-	P. S. Murthy best paper award, Association of Clinical Biochemists of India, India
2012-	Best poster award, Association of Clinical Biochemists of India, India
2012-2013	Indian Immunology Society (IIS) Bursary Award
2017-	University of Illinois College of Medicine Rockford recognition of scholarly contributions

Publications from the Last 3 Years:

1. Khatri V, Chauhan N, Kalyanasundaram R. Filarial parasite-derived new potential bio-therapeutic agents for inflammatory bowel diseases. *Adv Gastroenterol Hepatol Endoscopy*. 2019; 1(1): 1–5.
2. R Paul, M Ilamaran, V Khatri, N Amdare, MVR Reddy, P Kaliraj. Immunological evaluation of fusion protein of Brugia malayi abundant larval protein transcript-2 (BmALT-2) and Tuftsin in experimental mice model. *Parasite Epidemiol Control*. 2019; https://doi.org/10.1016/j.parepi.2019.e00092.
3. Khatri VK, Amdare N, Chauhan N, Togre N, Reddy MVR, Hoti SL, et al. Epidemiological screening and xenomonitoring of human Lymphatic Filariasis infection in select districts in the states of Maharashtra and Karnataka, *India. J Parasitol Res*. 2019; https://doi.org/10.1007/s00436-019-06205-0 (IF 2.558).
4. BV Siva Prasad, V Khatri, PS Yadav, MS Chandra, DV Lakshmi and K Goswami. Immunodiagnostic potential of Wuchereria bancrofti L1 antigen based filarial IgG4 detection assay. *Trans R Soc Trop Med Hyg*. 2018; 00:1-8. doi:10.1093/trstmh/try110 (IF 2.82).
5. Togre N, Khatri V, Nakhale M, Bhoj P, Goswami K, Tarnekar A, Patil M, Kumar S. Exploration of immune modulation by combination of filarial proteins against DSS induced acute colitis in mouse model. *Roum Arch Microbiol Immunol*. 2018; 77(2): 153-161.
6. Chauhan N*, Khatri VK*, Banerjee P, Kalyanasundaram R. Evaluating the vaccine potential of a tetravalent fusion protein (rBmHAXT) vaccine antigen against lymphatic filariasis in a mouse model. *Front. Immunol*. 2018; 9:1520. doi: 10.3389/fimmu.2018.01520. (IF 5.511).
   *Shared authorship.
7. Khatri VK, Chauhan N, Vishnoi K, Gegerfelt A, Gittens C, Kalyanasundaram R. Prospects of developing an effective

multivalent recombinant prophylactic vaccine against lymphatic filariasis – Evaluation of protection in non-human primates. *Int J Parasitol*. 2018; 48:773–783. https://doi.org/10.1016/j.ijpara. 2018.04.002 (IF 3.872).
8. Chauhan N, Banerjee P, Khatri VK, Canciamille A, Gilles J, Kalyanasundaram R. Improving the efficacy of a prophylactic vaccine formulation against lymphatic filariasis. *J Parasitol Res*. 2017 Aug 21:1-0. (IF: 2.558).
9. Ravi SP Yadav, V Khatri, Nitin Amdare, Kalyan Goswami, VB Shivkumar, Nitin Gangane, et al. Evaluation of preventive effect of Brugia malayi recombinant cystatin on antigen-induced experimental arthritis. *Indian J Exp Biol*. 2017; 55:655-660 (IF 1.475).
10. Togre NS, Bhoj PS, Khatri VK, Tarnekar A, Goswami K, Shende MR, et al. SXP–RAL Family Filarial Protein, rWbL2, Prevents Development of DSS-Induced Acute Ulcerative Colitis. *Indian J Clin Biochem*. 2017:1-8.
11. Immanuel C, Ramanathan A, Balasubramaniyan M, Khatri VK, Amdare NP, Rao DN, et al. Immunoprophylaxis of multi-antigen peptide (MAP) vaccine for human lymphatic filariasis. *Immunol Res*. 2017 Jun;65(3):729-738. (IF: 2.487).
12. Amdare NP, Khatri VK, Yadav RS, Tarnekar A, Goswami K, Reddy MV. Therapeutic potential of the immunomodulatory proteins *Wuchereria bancrofti* L2 and *Brugia malayi* abundant larval transcript 2 against streptozotocin-induced type 1 diabetes in mice. *J Helminthol*. 2016 Sep 26:1. (IF: 1.344)
13. Reddy SM, Reddy PM, Amdare N, Khatri V, Tarnekar A, Goswami K, et al. Filarial Abundant Larval Transcript Protein ALT-2: An Immunomodulatory Therapeutic Agent for Type 1 Diabetes. *Indian J Clin Biochem* 2016:1-8.
14. D Andure, K Pote, V Khatri, N Amdare, R Padalkar, MVR Reddy. Immunization with Wuchereria bancrofti glutathione-s-transferase elicits a mixed Th1/Th2 type of protective immune response

against filarial infection in mastomys. *Indian J Clin Biochem* 2016; doi:10.1007/s12291-016-0556-y.
15. Ravi SP Yadav, V Khatri, N Amdare, K Goswami, VB Shivkumar, N Gangane, et al. Immuno-modulatory effect and therapeutic potential of Brugia malayi cystatin in experimentally induced arthritis. *Indian J Clin Biochem* 2016 Apr;31(2):203-8.

INDEX

A

absorption capacity, 60
absorption of sulfate, 26, 27, 59
acid, 5, 25, 52, 56, 64, 72, 80, 81, 85, 91, 102, 103
active centers, 34
adaptive immune response, 78, 108
adaptive immune responses, 108
adenosine, 31, 65, 66
adenosine 5′-phosphosulfate (APS), 31, 32, 33, 35, 66
adenosine triphosphate, 65
adhesive properties, 54, 72
age, viii, 2, 5, 8, 9, 14, 15, 21, 39, 42, 55, 86
allergy, 77, 83, 94, 95, 100
amino acids, 21, 22, 27, 29, 33, 34, 59, 70
animal models of colitis, 41
animal studies, 81, 82, 83, 85, 89
antibiotic, vii, viii, ix, 2, 3, 5, 10, 11, 16
antibiotic treatment, vii, viii, ix, 2, 3, 5
antigen, 13, 14, 84, 85, 86, 87, 94, 102, 103, 104, 105, 110, 116, 122, 127, 128
apoptosis, 112, 123, 124, 125
arthritis, 79, 115, 122, 128, 129
assimilatory sulfate reduction, 21, 30, 33, 59

autoimmune disease, 96, 98

B

bacteria, vii, ix, 4, 6, 19, 20, 22, 23, 27, 28, 30, 32, 34, 36, 37, 38, 39, 40, 41, 43, 44, 46, 48, 52, 54, 55, 60, 62, 63, 64, 65, 66, 67, 68, 69, 70, 71, 72, 73, 83
bacterial cells, 31, 43
bacterium, 3, 87, 89
Bacteroides, 38, 44, 45, 46, 47, 55
beneficial effect, 96, 97
beverages, 21, 24, 26, 58, 60, 63
Bifidobacterium, 44, 45, 46, 47, 48, 54, 56, 57
biofilm, 38, 55, 61
bioinformatics, 125
biomarkers, 115
biomolecules, 92
biopsy, 39, 52, 55
biosynthesis, 70
bowel, vii, ix, 19, 20, 22, 27, 40, 45, 46, 47, 58, 59, 61, 100
breast cancer, 10, 116, 124
breast carcinoma, 106

Index

C

cabbage, 23, 25
caecum, 40, 49
calcium, 23, 24, 25, 26, 64
cancer, 26, 36, 37, 68, 96, 97
cell differentiation, 92
cephalosporin, 10, 15, 16
cephalosporin antibiotics, 16
chemically-induced models, 40, 57
children, vii, ix, 17, 39, 76
chronic colitis, 41, 89, 104, 105, 115, 117, 124
clinical diagnosis, 58
clinical studies, 82, 98
clinical trials, x, 76, 82, 83, 88, 95, 96, 97, 126
clostridium, v, vii, 1, 3, 4, 5, 6, 7, 9, 10, 15, 16, 17, 28, 38, 44, 45, 46, 47, 48, 54, 56, 58, 68
Clostridium, v, vii, 1, 3, 4, 5, 6, 7, 9, 10, 15, 16, 17, 28, 38, 44, 45, 46, 47, 48, 54, 56, 58, 68
clostridium difficile, v, vii, 1, 3, 4, 5, 6, 7, 9, 10, 15, 16, 17
colitis, vii, ix, 3, 14, 17, 37, 41, 42, 52, 53, 54, 55, 56, 57, 59, 60, 62, 63, 72, 73, 76, 79, 80, 81, 82, 83, 84, 85, 87, 88, 89, 90, 91, 92, 93, 94, 95, 96, 97, 98, 101, 102, 103, 104, 105, 107, 108, 109, 110, 111, 115, 116, 117, 118, 124, 125, 127
colon, 4, 10, 26, 27, 28, 29, 37, 38, 39, 41, 43, 44, 46, 47, 50, 51, 52, 53, 54, 56, 58, 59, 71, 72, 80, 87, 88, 89, 90, 91, 93
colon cancer, 10
colonic bacteria, 40, 52
colonization, 56, 58
colonoscopy, 70
colorectal cancer, 26
complications, x, 13, 16, 57, 76
composition, 39, 40, 41, 43, 47, 58, 61, 64
compounds, 25, 41, 48, 49, 50, 58, 59, 61, 72, 114, 115, 124
correlation, 21, 27, 50, 55, 63, 83
correlation analysis, 63
cysteine, 22, 27, 29, 30, 33, 86, 87, 94, 106, 107
cytokines, 80, 84, 87, 91, 92, 93, 94, 95
cytoplasm, 31, 33, 34

D

dendritic cell, 93, 94, 102, 111
descending colon, 49, 50, 53
Desulfovibrio, 20, 22, 31, 32, 33, 35, 36, 37, 38, 39, 40, 49, 59, 62, 63, 66, 67, 68, 69, 73
Desulfovibrio piger, 36, 62, 63, 67, 68, 73
detection, 7, 33, 45, 46, 47, 50, 51, 53, 54, 112, 116, 127
developed countries, ix, 20
development of IBD, 21, 22, 41, 54
diabetes, 5, 83, 92, 98, 110, 119
diabetes melitus, 5
diarrhea, viii, 2, 3, 4, 5, 6, 9, 12, 13, 14, 15, 16, 37, 54, 56, 72, 96
diet, ix, 19, 21, 22, 23, 26, 27, 29, 39, 42, 44, 45, 58, 59, 60
diseases, 5, 15, 21, 36, 37, 40, 41, 50, 57, 58, 59, 61, 79, 92, 99, 100
dissimilatory sulfate reduction, 21, 29, 30, 31, 32, 33, 35, 36, 59, 61, 62, 70
donors, 33, 34, 35, 70, 103
drinking water, 25, 26, 41
drug metabolism, 24
drugs, viii, 2, 5, 23, 56, 57, 97, 119

E

E. coli, 44, 45, 46, 47, 48, 54
educational research, 112

electron, ix, 19, 21, 28, 30, 32, 33, 34, 35, 39, 40, 50, 59, 67
electron acceptor, ix, 19, 21, 28, 30, 32, 33, 35, 39, 59
electron donor, ix, 19, 33, 34, 35, 39, 40
Enterobacteriacea, 43
environment, ix, 20, 25, 27, 32, 38, 83, 95
environmental conditions, 21
environmental stimuli, 77
enzyme, viii, 2, 7, 31, 32, 33, 88, 110
epidemiology, ix, 3, 17
epithelial cells, 52, 54
epithelium, 4, 26, 54
Escherichia, 28, 44, 54, 58, 67, 72, 73, 89
etiology, vii, ix, 19, 55, 56, 58, 98
evidence, vii, x, 55, 76, 86, 88
evolution, x, 15, 17, 76, 78, 99
excretion, 23, 27, 29, 63
exposure, 24, 52, 77, 78, 80, 83

F

fatty acids, 34, 39, 52
feces, vii, ix, 19, 26, 27, 33, 36, 37, 38, 49, 50, 52, 53, 54, 58, 59, 68
food, ix, 19, 21, 22, 23, 24, 25, 26, 41, 58, 59, 60, 61, 63, 64
food additive, 23, 59, 64
food products, 24, 61
formation, 4, 10, 31, 32, 33, 34, 35, 36, 53, 58, 64, 86
fruits, ix, 19, 21, 23, 24, 26
fusion, 122, 126, 127

G

gastrointestinal tract, 27, 29, 36, 39, 45, 57, 58, 69, 70
genes, 32, 33, 65, 67, 77, 78, 99, 100
genetic diversity, 99
genetic factors, 98

genetic information, 57
genetic predisposition, 21, 77, 100
genus, viii, ix, 2, 19, 22, 31, 32, 33, 36, 37, 38, 39, 40, 43, 47, 59, 68, 93
glutathione, 95, 109, 122, 128
glycoproteins, 26, 29, 84
growth, 36, 39, 40, 44, 59, 61, 62, 63, 69, 71
guidelines, 17, 83

H

health, x, 3, 14, 22, 27, 57, 61, 64, 65, 76
helminth therapy, v, 75, 76, 79, 82, 83, 92, 104
human, 21, 22, 26, 29, 36, 37, 38, 39, 40, 41, 43, 52, 57, 58, 59, 61, 65, 68, 69, 70, 78, 79, 82, 83, 92, 94, 95, 97, 98, 99, 100, 106, 112, 114, 118, 120, 121, 126, 127, 128
human body, 29, 39
human gastrointestinal tract, 29, 39, 69, 70
hydrogen, ix, 20, 21, 22, 26, 27, 28, 30, 32, 33, 34, 35, 36, 38, 39, 40, 48, 53, 58, 59, 60, 61, 63, 64, 65, 67, 71
hydrogen sulfide, ix, 20, 21, 22, 26, 27, 28, 30, 32, 33, 35, 36, 38, 40, 48, 50, 52, 53, 58, 59, 60, 61, 63, 71
hydrogenase, 34, 66, 67
hygiene, ix, 3, 16, 78, 99, 100
hygiene hypothesis, 77, 78, 99, 100
hyperplasia, 37, 52
hypertrophy, 110
hypothesis, 78, 99, 100

I

IFN, 81, 84, 85, 88, 90, 91, 93
IL-13, 84, 88, 90, 95
IL-17, 84, 85, 88, 93, 101
immune function, 78

immune modulation, 99, 112, 116, 118, 124, 127
immune reaction, 92
immune regulation, 92, 100
immune response, x, 41, 76, 77, 79, 80, 86, 88, 93, 105, 109, 123, 128
immune system, 55, 77, 83, 86, 87, 88, 94, 98
immunocompromised, vii, viii, 2, 9, 69
immunogenicity, 88, 95
immunomodulation, 79, 96, 109
immunomodulator, 106, 107, 110
immunomodulatory, x, 76, 79, 83, 86, 87, 88, 93, 94, 96, 98, 108, 113, 114, 122, 128
in vitro, 94, 104, 109, 114, 125
in vivo, 94
incidence, vii, viii, ix, 2, 3, 5, 6, 8, 9, 10, 15, 16, 20, 56, 62, 76, 77
infection, 3, 4, 11, 13, 15, 16, 17, 37, 70, 78, 80, 82, 88, 93, 95, 99, 100, 101, 102, 103, 118, 121, 123, 127, 129
inflammation, 12, 41, 42, 54, 55, 73, 80, 81, 89, 93, 95, 102, 104, 107, 108, 109, 110, 111
inflammatory bowel disease (IBD), vii, ix, 2, 19, 20, 21, 22, 36, 40, 41, 52, 53, 54, 56, 57, 58, 59, 61, 62, 68, 70, 71, 72, 73, 76, 79, 82, 84, 92, 94, 96, 97, 100, 101, 103, 107, 111, 127
Inflammatory bowel disease (IBD), ix, 19, 20
inhibition, 17, 32, 36, 52, 60, 72, 86, 116, 124
interferon, 81, 85, 91
interferon-γ, 81, 85, 91
internal environment, 14
intestinal absorption, 29, 59
intestine, 4, 14, 29, 30, 33, 34, 35, 36, 37, 39, 40, 41, 51, 53, 59, 60, 65, 68, 93, 101, 102, 110
ion transport, 80, 81, 101

ions, 31, 39, 45, 59

K

Klebsiella, 44, 45, 46, 47, 48, 54, 58, 72

L

lactic acid, 34, 60
Lactobacillus, 44, 45, 46, 47, 48, 54, 56, 57
large intestine, 34, 43, 48, 49, 51, 52, 65, 68, 69
lumen, 22, 33, 35, 39, 40, 43, 47, 54, 58, 59, 61
lumen microbiota, 43
lymph node, 92
lymphoma, 10, 96, 111

M

macrophages, 81, 87, 88, 89, 90, 91, 93, 94, 95, 107, 109, 111
metabolic syndrome, 112, 115
metabolism, ix, 20, 24, 26, 30, 36, 40, 52, 57, 65, 67, 69, 112, 123, 125
mice, 41, 55, 62, 73, 80, 84, 87, 88, 89, 92, 93, 94, 95, 101, 102, 103, 104, 105, 106, 107, 108, 110, 111, 114, 115, 120, 122, 124, 127, 128
microbiota, 36, 41, 43, 44, 45, 46, 47, 48, 54, 55, 57, 58, 60, 68, 70
microorganisms, 21, 32, 34, 38, 39, 43, 45, 46, 47, 54, 57, 59, 60, 65, 68
microparticles, 109
molecular hydrogen, 33, 34, 36, 39, 40
molecular mass, 85
molecular mimicry, 95
molecular weight, 31, 32
molecules, 23, 34, 55, 77, 79, 83, 84, 86, 87, 88, 92, 96, 97, 120

Index

mortality, ix, 3, 11, 16, 20, 21
mucosa, 4, 22, 29, 38, 39, 41, 50, 52, 54, 56, 70, 71
myocardial infarction, 13

N

nematode, 101, 105, 106, 110, 111
neuroendocrine system, 39
nutrition, 22, 39, 41, 43, 64, 72

O

organic compounds, ix, 19, 30, 34, 35, 39, 40, 49, 59
oxidation, 27, 29, 33, 34, 35, 49, 52, 66, 71, 72

P

parasite, 78, 79, 86, 87, 88, 97, 99, 102, 105, 107, 108, 112, 114, 115, 116, 119, 124, 125, 127
parasitic diseases, vii, x, 76
pathogenesis, 36, 52, 54, 55, 56, 57, 61, 70, 112
pathology, 87, 89, 90, 105
pathophysiological, 112
pathophysiology, 27, 56
periplasmic hydrogenases, 34
phenotype, 77, 79, 87, 108
polymerase chain reaction, 70
population, 10, 12, 21, 22, 23, 24, 44, 62, 77
population group, 23
positive correlation, 25, 50
postgate medium, 43
prevention of infection, 16
probiotic, 5, 89, 98, 107
prognosis, ix, 3, 14, 16
pro-inflammatory, 93, 95

proliferation, 52, 81, 93, 106
protease inhibitors, 87, 89, 90, 94
protection, 81, 83, 85, 93, 94, 98, 102, 110, 126, 128
proteins, x, 21, 23, 34, 67, 76, 78, 84, 85, 87, 88, 94, 97, 98, 104, 105, 113, 114, 115, 116, 117, 118, 119, 122, 124, 127, 128
Proteus, 44, 45, 46, 47, 48, 54, 58
pyogenic, 37, 38
pyogenic liver, 37, 38
pyogenic liver abscess, 37, 38
pyrophosphate, 31

R

receptor, 81, 91, 108, 111, 116
recombinant proteins, 76, 86, 89, 98, 117, 119, 120
recurrence, viii, 2, 3, 14, 16
relapses, viii, ix, 2, 3, 12, 82
response, 55, 77, 79, 81, 85, 86, 92, 95, 109, 116, 124
rheumatic diseases, 36
rheumatoid arthritis, 84, 106, 112, 125
risk, viii, 2, 3, 4, 6, 11, 12, 13, 14, 15, 16, 57, 80, 96, 97
risk factors, viii, 2, 3, 4, 6, 9, 11, 16

S

safety, 83, 86, 88, 95, 97, 104
side effects, vii, x, 5, 76, 82, 96
sodium, 23, 24, 25, 31, 41, 43, 52, 64, 65, 80, 81, 85, 91, 101, 105, 108
source of sulfate, 24, 25, 26, 27, 29, 39, 58
species, ix, 19, 22, 31, 32, 35, 36, 37, 38, 39, 40, 54, 55, 59, 63, 68, 78, 80
Staphylococcus, 44, 45, 46, 47, 48, 54, 58
sulfate, v, vii, ix, 19, 20, 21, 22, 23, 24, 25, 26, 27, 28, 29, 30, 31, 32, 33, 35, 36, 39,

40, 41, 43, 45, 48, 49, 54, 55, 57, 58, 59, 60, 61, 62, 63, 64, 65, 66, 67, 68, 69, 70, 71, 73, 80, 81, 85, 91, 101, 105, 108
sulfate concentrations, 23, 25
sulfate content, 21, 22, 24, 25, 26, 27, 29, 41, 58
sulfate in food, 22, 59, 60, 63
sulfate in the colon, 28
sulfate reduction process, 21, 29, 33, 59
sulfate secretion, 29
sulfate-containing medium, 22, 59
sulfate-reducing bacteria (SRB), vii, ix, 19, 20, 21, 22, 23, 26, 27, 28, 29, 30, 31, 32, 33, 34, 35, 36, 37, 38, 39, 40, 41, 43, 44, 45, 46, 47, 48, 49, 52, 53, 54, 57, 58, 59, 60, 61, 62, 63, 65, 66, 67, 68, 69, 70, 71, 73
sulfite, ix, 20, 23, 24, 25, 32, 33, 59, 64, 66
sulfite reductase, 32, 33, 66
sulfonamide, 10, 115, 124
sulfur, 23, 24, 27, 29, 30, 32, 33, 48, 59, 63, 66, 71, 72
suppression, 5, 80, 87, 88, 89, 90, 93, 108
symptoms, viii, 2, 4, 10, 11, 16, 41, 81, 88, 91
synthesis, 21, 22, 30, 33, 59, 94, 95

T

T cell, 80, 81, 84, 85, 87, 88, 92, 93, 94, 96, 101, 102, 105, 106, 107, 111, 120
target, 17, 94, 112
therapeutic agents, 127
therapeutic approaches, 96
therapeutic effect, 80, 83, 84, 125
therapeutic effects, 80, 83
therapeutics, x, 76, 83, 92, 96, 98, 120, 125
therapy, viii, ix, x, 2, 3, 5, 10, 11, 14, 16, 61, 70, 76, 79, 81, 82, 83, 94, 96, 97, 98, 101, 103, 111, 112

TNF-α, 80, 81, 84, 85, 88, 90, 91, 93, 95, 96, 116
toxic effect, 36
toxic megacolon, 3
toxicity, 52, 71
toxin, vii, viii, 1, 2, 4, 7, 8, 9, 13, 14, 15, 64
treatment, vii, viii, ix, 2, 3, 4, 5, 9, 13, 14, 15, 16, 17, 25, 40, 56, 80, 83, 84, 87, 90, 91, 96, 97, 103, 107, 108, 111, 119, 125
tumor necrosis factor, 81, 85, 91
type 1 diabetes, 79, 84, 114, 119, 122, 125, 128

U

ulcerations, 4, 52, 53, 58
ulcerative colitis, vii, ix, x, 9, 19, 20, 37, 41, 42, 53, 54, 55, 56, 62, 63, 64, 65, 69, 70, 71, 72, 73, 76, 82, 103, 111, 113, 115, 118, 122, 124, 128

V

vaccine, 88, 122, 125, 126, 127, 128

W

water quality, 64
weight loss, 13, 14, 37, 88, 89, 90
whole worm therapy, 79, 81
worms, x, 76, 83, 96, 101

Related Nova Publications

DIVERTICULAR DISEASE: COLONIC EPIDEMY OF THE 21ST CENTURY

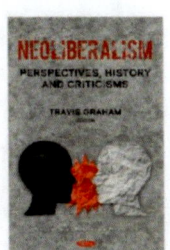

EDITORS: Andrés García-Marín, MD, PhD and Jaime Ruiz-Tovar, MD, PhD

SERIES: Digestive Diseases – Research and Clinical Developments

BOOK DESCRIPTION: Diverticular disease is one of the most common problems encountered by gastroenterologists, emergency physicians and surgeons, with a higher prevalence in elderly patients and a dramatic rising of incidences in young people, which involve an increase in health care costs, according to ambulatory visits and hospital admissions. The aim of this book is to revise the current evidence about the diverticular disease and acute diverticulitis.

SOFTCOVER ISBN: 978-1-53615-989-9
RETAIL PRICE: $82

FLAVONOIDS IN THE FIGHT AGAINST UPPER GASTROINTESTINAL TRACT CANCERS

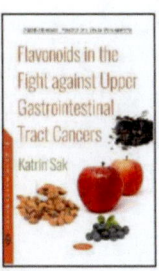

AUTHOR: Katrin Sak

SERIES: Digestive Diseases – Research and Clinical Developments

BOOK DESCRIPTION: This book gives a comprehensive and contemporary survey about the different anticancer actions of various natural and semisynthetic flavonoids in experimental models of oral, pharyngeal, esophageal and gastric cancers, involving the data obtained from studies of both cell lines as well as laboratorial animals.

HARDCOVER ISBN: 978-1-53613-570-1
RETAIL PRICE: $230

To see a complete list of Nova publications, please visit our website at www.novapublishers.com

Related Nova Publications

Lecture Notes on Pancreatitis

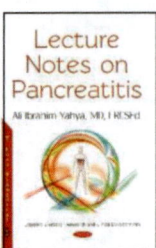

Author: Ali Ibrahim Yahya, M.D.

Series: Digestive Diseases – Research and Clinical Developments

Book Description: This book covers topics of pancreatitis including pathology, clinical presentation, investigations and treatment; it is recommended for resident surgeons and will help them to attain knowledge on pancreatitis.

Softcover ISBN: 978-1-53613-034-8
Retail Price: $82

Dysphagia: Complications, Management and Clinical Aspects

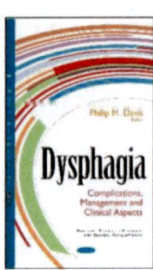

Editor: Philip M. Davis

Series: Digestive Diseases – Research and Clinical Developments

Book Description: Dysphagia is the difficulty or improper swallowing of liquids, solids, or even saliva. This book provides new research on the complications, management and clinical aspects of dysphagia.

Hardcover ISBN: 978-1-53610-432-5
Retail Price: $95

To see a complete list of Nova publications, please visit our website at www.novapublishers.com